FINAL FRCA: THE SHORT ANSWER QUESTIONS

FINAL FRCA: THE SHORT ANSWER QUESTIONS

James Nickells
Specialist Registrar in Anaesthesia

Maan Hasan
Consultant Anaesthetist

Vino Ramachandra
Consultant Anaesthetist

Neville Robinson
Consultant Anaesthetist

Department of Anaesthesia, Northwick Park and St Mark's Hospitals, Harrow, Middlesex, UK.

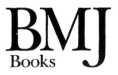
BMJ Books

First published in 1998
Second impression 2002
by BMJ Books, BMA House, Tavistock Square,
London WC1H 9JR

British Library Cataloguing in Publication Data

A catalogue record for this book is available from the British Library

ISBN 0–7279–1289–5

Typeset by Apek Typesetters, Nailsea, Bristol
Printed and bound by Selwood Priting Ltd. West Sussex

Contents

Introduction–Advice on answering questions   1

Paper A
    Questions   4
    Answers   5

Paper B
    Questions   22
    Answers   23

Paper C
    Questions   39
    Answers   40

Paper D
    Questions   55
    Answers   56

Paper E
    Questions   73
    Answers   74

Paper F
    Questions   88
    Answers   89

Paper G
    Questions   105
    Answers   106

Paper H
    Questions   125
    Answers   126

Paper I
    Questions   142
    Answers   143

Index by key words   159

Introduction–Advice on answering questions

The "Short Answer Questions" section of the final examination for the Fellowship of the Royal College of Anaesthetists comprises of 12 compulsory questions which must be answered in three hours. This small book puts together nine examination papers for prospective candidates to practise from. These examination standard questions are designed to test a candidate's knowledge of the whole syllabus and include what we consider to be ideal answers.

As this book has been written we have listened to the problems that successful and unsuccessful examination candidates have told us about what they have experienced. These are recounted below.

The most important issue is "breadth of knowledge" relating to all aspects of the practice and principles of anaesthesia. The syllabus is widely available and does not need repetition here. If a question cannot be attempted the candidate is obviously placed at a considerable disadvantage! Widespread general knowledge is mandatory and unsuccessful candidates inform us that gaps in a specific area are always discovered in some aspect of the examination.

All the questions are equally "weighted", and this therefore leads us to the biggest problem that the candidates have in the examination. This is the "time factor". All questions have an equal time allocation and there is no benefit to be derived from spending extra time completing one answer at the expense of an incomplete brief answer to another question. Answers must be precise.

The examination is 180 minutes in duration and it takes at least 5–10 minutes at the start to read the questions and commence the first answer. We consider that at the end of the examination a further 10 minutes are needed to read and correct your answers to each question. This is only 50 seconds per question. There is a big advantage in this. It means that the candidate is not writing the last answer under huge self-inflicted pressure when there are many distractions. Each answer should take no longer than 14 minutes and this rule must be rigidly adhered to throughout each answer. No answer can take longer than 14 minutes! This includes working out the structure to the answer so in fact most answers have to be written

1

in about 12 minutes actual time. Some of the questions appear to need answers longer than this in duration so in these cases only the major aspects of the subject can be alluded to. We estimate that no answer can be longer than 300 words and have tried to keep to this rule when doing our "model" answers.

The answers must be answered in accordance with the style of the question. Read the question carefully! There are a variety of question styles:

- "Choice of anaesthesia for. . ."
- "Outline with reasons the anaesthetic. . ."
- "List with reasons. . ."
- "List the most important. . ."
- "Write a letter to a general practitioner. . ."
- "Write a medical report. . ."

Answer in an appropriate manner! A letter or a medical report means that the answer must be in sentenced, paragraphed style. A list means precisely that and nothing more. Anaesthesia can be performed under general or regional techniques and, if reasons are requested, it means the advantages and disadvantages of each technique are required.

Structured answers are advantageous. Clinical subjects can often be specifically answered using pre-, intra-, and postoperative headings. Regional anaesthetic questions can often be answered by an answer that includes indications, contraindications, resuscitation equipment, consent, sterility, patient position, surface anatomy, needle type and passage, solution injected, complications and recovery. Drawings should be large, clearly labelled and referred to in the text. A clear "line" drawing is often acceptable. An unexplained figure is meaningless!

The candidate must understand how the examination is marked. A basic answer with most of the correct matters mentioned will pass. Glaring omissions will fail a candidate and so the first and most important consideration is to get "core facts" down on paper in an orderly fashion. The examiners, after reading a paper, know who has enough knowledge to pass. They are also looking for the 2+ paper and this candidate will have inserted better knowledge into the text. He or she will have consistently higher standards of basic facts written down, but will have shown that there are areas of debate or controversy about some of the subjects and will have shown, after the basic answer is written, a knowledge in greater depth than other candidates.

It is hardly necessary to write down the following but, without clarity of written expression, it is difficult to pass. Therefore:

- Be punctual.
- Don't be distracted.
- Write clearly.
- Write legibly.

2

- Spell correctly.
- Read the question.
- Answer the question.
- Space answers well.
- Make drawings big.
- Label figures.
- Structure answers.
- Know "definitions".
- Put basic facts first.
- Anatomy knowledge is essential.
- In-depth knowledge is necessary only if time allows.
- Stay strictly to time.
- Practise answers.

This book is designed to give the candidate some examination practice. The book has been carefully structured so that either whole examinations can be completed or a number of questions relating to one topic, for example obstetrics, can be attempted. The list of the "key words" appears at the back of the book and we feel that this may help candidates who are wishing to practise answers on a specific topic. The "key word" to each question is also at the bottom of each page and this helps in selecting a specific question to practise. There are many ways of answering questions correctly using different "styles of answer" and to this end we have deliberately answered questions in a variety of suitable styles which are likely to be acceptable to the examiner. We have even provided similar but different questions on a specific topic to illustrate how apparently similar questions require quite different answers.

Good luck! Everyone needs some!

Paper A

1. Define pregnancy-induced hypertension. List the maternal complications of the condition.

2. Write short notes on (a) parametric and non-parametric tests, and (b) statistical probability.

3. Write a short account on porphyria. List the drugs used in anaesthetic practice that may precipitate an acute attack.

4. Discuss the problems of general anaesthesia in a morbidly obese patient.

5. Write notes on the techniques available for decontamination, disinfection, and sterilisation of soiled theatre equipment.

6. Outline the chronic pain management of a 35 year-old patient who has a solitary rib metastasis from a primary breast carcinoma.

7. What are the main objectives of care in the recovery unit? List the main criteria for discharge of a patient from the recovery unit.

8. Write a short essay on ankylosing spondylitis with special reference to anaesthesia.

9. Describe the important tracheal relations. List the indications for tracheostomy.

10. Define medical audit. Write short notes on (a) the NCEPOD and, (b) the confidential enquiries into maternal deaths.

11. List the indications, contraindications, and complications of stellate ganglion block.

12. Outiine the advantages and disadvantages of performing a transurethral resection of the prostate (TURP) using regional anaesthesia rather than general anaesthesia.

1. Define pregnancy-induced hypertension. List the maternal complications of the condition.

Pregnancy-induced hypertension (PIH) is difficult to define. The International Society for the Study of Hypertension in Pregnancy defines PIH as a single diastolic reading (phase V) of ≥ 110 mmHg or above, or two readings of ≥ 90 mmHg or greater at least four hours apart, occurring after the 20th week of pregnancy in a previously normotensive woman. An American Working Group has defined it as a rise of > 15 mmHg diastolic or > 30 mmHg systolic compared with readings taken earlier in pregnancy (this definition allows for the identification of women with PIH that is superimposed on chronic hypertension).

A diastolic pressure of > 90 mmHg before 20 weeks suggests chronic hypertension. While oedema and proteinuria are not essential for the diagnosis, proteinuria remains a hallmark of the severity of this disorder. Proteinuria is defined as a $2+$ strip test on two occasions four hours apart or a 24-hour collection with a total protein of > 0.3 g. Eclampsia is an extreme hypertensive disorder of pregnancy and is defined as a generalised convulsion occurring during pregnancy, labour, or within seven days of delivery in the absence of epilepsy or any other disorder predisposing to convulsions.

The complications are multisystemic and are listed below:

- *Placenta*–abruptio placenta, intrauterine growth retardation
- *Cerebral*–hyperreflexia/clonus, convulsions, visual disturbances, cerebral haemorrhage
- *Renal*–proteinuria, renal failure
- *Hepatic*–liver dysfunction (HELLP - haemolysis, elevated liver enzymes, low platelets), periportal necrosis, subcapsular haematoma, epigastric pain
- *Haematological*–thrombocytopenia, haemolysis, disseminated intravascular coagulation
- *Cardiovascular*–hypovolaemia, abnormal left ventricular function, pulmonary oedema.

KEYWORDS: PREGNANCY-INDUCED HYPERTENSION

2. Write short notes on (a) parametric and non-parametric tests, and (b) statistical probability.

(a) Parametric and non-parametric tests

These tests of inferential statistics (as opposed to descriptive statistics) are designed to draw conclusions regarding differences between two or more sets of data.

Parametric tests are used when the following two basic requirements are met. Firstly, the data are of the interval, continuous, or ratio type, and secondly, the data are normally distributed. Examples include the application of Student's t test when two groups of data are involved, or the analysis of variance (ANOVA) when there are more than two groups of data.

Non-parametric tests are also called distribution-free statistical tests. These tests are suitable for ordinal data, such as in Wilcoxon rank tests, or nominal data such as in chi-square test. They are also used for interval, continuous, or ratios data that are *not* normally distributed, such as in Mann–Whitney U test when two groups of data are studied, or Kruskal–Wallis when more than two groups of data are involved.

(b) Statistical probability

This is a number ≥ 0 and ≤ 1 or ratio expressing the numerical likelihood of occurrence of an event. It represents the ratio of the number of actual occurrences to the number of possible occurrences. A probability outcome in a statistical test of $P < 0.05$ is usually taken as significant. This represents an acceptance as significant any null hypothesis event that occurs less frequently than once in 20 times. The level of probability determines the frequency with which type I (or type a) and type II (or type b) errors occur. Type I occurs when one erroneously concludes that a difference exists when there is no real difference. Alternatively, type II error occurs when one is not able to detect any difference between groups of data when a difference really exists. A common cause for the latter error is insufficient sample size which can be avoided by performing power analysis.

KEYWORDS: PARAMETRIC/NON-PARAMETRIC TESTS; PROBABILITY; STATISTICS

3. Write a short account on porphyria. List the drugs used in anaesthetic practice that may precipitate an acute attack.

The porphyrias are an inherited group of metabolic, autosomally-linked genetic disorders of porphyrin metabolism. They are characterised by lack or partial block of the functional enzymes in the biosynthetic pathway of haem. This causes an overproduction of porphyrins. Porphyria is classified into the acute porphyrias which include intermittent porphyria and variegate porphyria, and the non-acute porphyrias which include porphyria cutanea tarda and erythropoietic porphyria.

Acute attacks of porphyria may be precipitated by triggers such as infection, administration of drugs (see list below), fasting, or menstruation. These attacks usually present with nausea, vomiting, acute abdominal pain, and variable degrees of neurological dysfunction. These include lower motor neurone lesions leading to paralysis and loss of sensation of a limb or bulbar palsy, peripheral neuropathy, and/or autonomic dysfunction. Mental disturbances, coma, convulsions and cranial nerve palsies have all been described. During the acute attack, the colour of the urine is typically described as dark brown on standing or red fluorescent under ultraviolet light. The appearance of aminolaevulinic acid in urine and porphyrins in the faeces are characteristic of acute intermittent porphyria and acute variegate porphyria respectively.

Drugs that may precipitate acute attacks of porphyria are listed under the two categories below.

(1) *High-risk precipitants* (should never be given)
All barbiturates, especially thiopentone
Chlordiazepoxide
Phenytoin
Meprobamate
Sulfonamides
Chloramphenicol

(2) *Unpredictable and controversial drugs* (should be avoided when possible)
Hyoscine
Metoclopromide
Chloral hydrate
Diazepam, but not temazepam which is known to be safe
Halothane and enflurane
Alcuronium
Lignocaine
Cocaine

KEYWORDS: PORPHYRIA

Non-steroidal anti-inflammatory drugs, namely diclofenac, mefenamic acid, and piroxicam

Angiotensin-converting enzyme inhibitors such as captopril, enalapril, and lisinopril

Clonidine

Hydralazine

Amiodarone

Ergot preparations

NB. Quite modest changes in the chemical structure of drugs of the same group change their porphyrinogenicity.

KEYWORDS: PORPHYRIA

4. Discuss the problems of general anaesthesia in a morbidly obese patient.

The problems of general anaesthesia in such a patient are the result of:

- pathophysiological changes
- concurrent disorders
- alterations in drug metabolism
- physical effects of morbid obesity

Preoperative problems

- *Cardiovascular derangements*–cardiac output and blood volume are increased; systemic hypertension is common; pulmonary hypertension is present in Pickwickian patients; left and right ventricular hypertrophy and biventricular failure; higher incidence of ischaemic heart disease.
- *Respiratory changes*–obesity is accompanied by hypoxaemia due to increased oxygen consumption, reduced pulmonary compliance, increased work of breathing, decreased FRC, ventilation-perfusion mismatch.
- *Gastrointestinal derangements*–higher incidence of gastro-oesophageal reflux and hiatus hernia; increased risk of pulmonary aspiration.
- *Associated conditions*–endocrine disorders, obstructive sleep apnoea, Pickwickian syndrome.

Intraoperative problems

The following are often difficult:

- Veins to find and cannulate.
- Airway maintenance with face mask; tracheal intubation–short neck, large breasts, rapid sequence induction.
- Blood pressure measurement.
- Lifting and positioning.
- Surgical access.
- Regional techniques.
- Drugs–lipophylic drugs such as opioids, benzodiazepines, and barbiturates have an increased volume of distribution and decreased elimination half-life (exception fentanyl); obesity increases the biotransformation rate of enflurane and halothane resulting in increased serum levels of fluoride ions; neuromuscular blocking agents should be given according to lean body weight.

KEYWORDS: OBESITY

Postoperative problems

- Atelectasis and hypoventilation are common with increased risk of hypoxaemia, infection and respiratory failure; elective IPPV may be required.
- Increased incidence of DVT–subcutaneous heparin and early ambulation required.
- Good pain control important for both improved pulmonary function and early ambulation.
- Wound dehiscence.

KEYWORDS: OBESITY

5. Write notes on the techniques available for decontamination, disinfection, and sterilisation of soiled theatre equipment.

Decontamination

This is defined as the removal of organic matter from equipment. It does not involve the killing of either bacteria or spores. It has a decreasing role in the modern medical environment with increased concern about cross-infection and the rise in use of disposable equipment.

Disinfection

Disinfection involves the killing of vegetative organisms, but does not affect all bacterial or fungal spores or viruses. Various methods are used to disinfect equipment:

- *Pasteurisation*–this involves heating in hot, but not boiling, water (usually 80°C for 10 minutes).
- *Boiling*–this is a more efficient technique and requires less time than pasteurisation. It is important to monitor the temperature to ensure high enough temperatures.
- *Chlorhexidine*–this is a non-detergent disinfectant that is mixed with aqueous or alcoholic solutions of different concentrations. It does not damage rubber.
- *Gluteraldehyde*–this is an expensive disinfectant which, if used for extended periods of time, also has some antispore activity. It is mixed with an activator and then has to be used within 14 days. Residual gluteraldehyde can cause pulmonary oedema. It is therefore important that it is washed off after use. Gluteraldehyde is commonly used in the disinfection of endoscopic equipment.
- *Sodium hypochlorite*–this has good activity against viruses but corrodes metal. It is generally used as a surface disinfectant to clean floors and walls in theatre.
- *70% alcohol.*
- *Phenolic compounds.*

Sterilisation

Sterilisation implies the killing of all micro-organisms, including spores and viruses.

- *Autoclaving*–this is a term used to define the application of steam and pressure to equipment. It is suitable for a wide range of equipment, including metal, cloth, glass, and some thermoresistant plastics. It may

KEYWORDS: STERILISATION OF EQUIPMENT; DECONTAMINATION; DISINFECTION; EQUIPMENT, STERILISATION

11

cause some plastics to degrade with repeated use.
- *Ethylene oxide*–gaseous ethylene oxide at a humidity of 30–40% acts as an alkylating agent to kill micro-organisms. It is a useful technique for the sterilisation of anaesthetic machines and electronic equipment. At the end of the sterilisation phase, an aeration phase is required to remove toxic residues from the equipment. This can make this technique time-consuming.
- *Formaldehyde sterilisation.*
- *Radiosterilisation.*

KEYWORDS: STERILISATION OF EQUIPMENT; DECONTAMINATION; DISINFECTION; EQUIPMENT, STERILISATION

6. Outline the chronic pain management of a 35 year-old patient who has a solitary rib metastasis from a primary breast carcinoma.

Care is multidisciplinary and involves surgeons, oncologists, chronic pain teams including specialist nurses, and importantly the patient and his or her family. The management of this patient is not the same as managing a terminally ill patient and the patient will probably want an active lifestyle. An assessment as to whether treatment should be instituted on an inpatient or an outpatient basis must be made.

Pain is subjective and treatment with minimal side effects should be aimed for. Pain management is likely at this stage to be of a short-term nature since the definitive treatment will probably involve radiotherapy to obliterate the secondary lesion.

An empathic approach and regular counselling of the patient is essential. *Drug treatment* involves options ranging from simple oral analgesics to opiates given orally or systemically, for example via subcutaneous syringe drivers. Opiate addiction in short-term therapy is not a major problem but nausea, vomiting, and constipation can be troublesome. Antidepressants and antiepileptic drugs have been used with limited success.

Regional blocks are not really suitable in this situation although intercostal nerve blocks may be helpful. These can be given intermittently or via an indwelling catheter but are likely only to provide short-term relief. In the terminally ill patient thoracic epidural infusions can be inserted with a view to long-term care but are unlikely to be of use in this situation.

Complementary medical therapies include TNS machines and acupuncture, and these have a role in management. They are associated with minimal side effects.

Regular follow-up even on a daily basis may be needed, even in the outpatient situation, in order to ensure that the situation does not deteriorate.

KEYWORDS: CHRONIC PAIN MANAGEMENT; RIB METASTASIS; BREAST CARCINOMA

7. What are the main objectives of care in the recovery unit? List the main criteria for discharge of a patient from the recovery unit.

Specialised recovery staff care for the patient ideally on a one-to-one basis after anaesthesia but the overall responsibility of patient care remains with the anaesthetist.

The *objectives of care* are as follows:

- Management of the airway.
- Assessment and management of the unconscious patient.
- Pain relief management, including the management of epidural devices.
- Observation of the patient.
- Clinical and technical monitoring as indicated – non-invasive blood pressure measurement, pulse, temperature, and oximetry are mandatory; however, in more complex cases, invasive monitoring is necessary.
- Management of shivering.
- Management of hypothermia.
- Management of nausea and vomiting.
- Care of intravenous infusions.
- Oxygen therapy.
- Observation of urine output.
- Observation of surgical wounds.

The *discharge criteria* include:

- Awake patient.
- Patient responds appropriately to commands.
- Patent upper airway.
- Airway reflexes present.
- Satisfactory respiration.
- Cardiovascular stability.
- Control of vomiting.
- Adequate pain control.

KEYWORDS: RECOVERY UNIT CARE; DISCHARGE FROM RECOVERY UNIT

8. Write a short essay on ankylosing spondylitis with special reference to anaesthesia.

Ankylosing spondylitis is a chronic inflammatory disease of unknown origin, commonest in young males, and characterised by progressive ossification of ligaments, joint cartilages, and disc spaces of the axial skeleton, with eventual fusion (ankylosis) of the spine and its adjacent structures. In extreme cases the patient develops a characteristic forward flexion of the spine, called a "poker spine" or "bamboo" spine.

Cervical and airway problems

Cervical spine spondylitis, arthrodesis, and involvement of the temporo-mandibular joints result in a progressive increase in the rigidity of the cervical vertebrae with limitation of neck movements. This also increases cervical instability with increased risk of atlanto-axial subluxation or cervical spine fractures.

Respiratory and cardiac problems

Involvement of the costovertebral joints with kyphoscoliosis causes rigidity of the thoracic cage. This is usually coupled with impaired lung function caused by pulmonary fibrosis, a common association with this disease. These changes result in severe restrictive type of lung function disorder. Cardiac involvements are rare. Examples of lesions reported are aortic regurgitation, cardiomyopathy, and bundle branch block.

Anaesthesia

General anaesthesia carries risks of difficulty in the management of the airway and tracheal intubation. Awake fibreoptic intubation is therefore frequently recommended. The risks of cervical (bony or neurological) injury require careful positioning of the head and neck on the table, especially when the patient is unconscious. The fixed thoracic cage and the fibrosis of the lungs increase the risk of postoperative respiratory complications (atelectasis and inability to cough efficiently to clear secretions). Regional (epidural or spinal) anaesthesia avoids many of these problems but it is usually technically difficult and sometimes impossible because of the fusion of the vertebral column. Caudal anaesthesia may be used as the sacral hiatus is commonly unfused.

KEYWORDS: ANKYLOSING SPONDYLITIS

9. Describe the important tracheal relations. List the indications for tracheostomy.

Tracheal relations

The trachea originates at the cricoid (C6 level) and terminates at the carina (T4 level). In the cervical part of its course the trachea lies in the mid-line, but within the thorax it is deviated slightly to the right by the arch of the aorta.

Relations in the neck
- anteriorly–skin, superficial and deep fascia, anterior jugular arch, strap muscles, isthmus of thyroid (2nd–4th rings), pretracheal fascia, brachio-cephalic artery, left brachiocephalic vein, arch of aorta
- posteriorly–oesophagus and recurrent laryngeal nerves
- laterally–carotid sheath and thyroid lobes.

These relations are outlined in the drawing below.

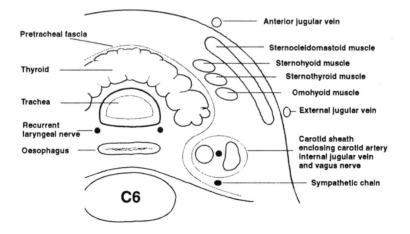

Relations in the chest
- anteriorly–inferior thyroid veins, origins of sternothyroid muscles from the back of the manubrium, remains of thymus
- on the right lie the pleura and lung with the superior vena cava
- on the left, the aortic arch and left vagus intervene between the trachea and pleura.

Indications for tracheostomy

Emergency
- relief of upper airway obstruction

KEYWORDS: TRACHEA, ANATOMY; TRACHEOSTOMY

Elective
- aid weaning from mechanical ventilation
- facilitate tracheobronchial toilet
- protect against aspiration of saliva and gastric contents, for example in chronic neurological disease
- laryngectomy for cancer
- major head and neck surgery–as a planned procedure to secure the airway in the postoperative period
- in children, to secure the airway in the presence of congenital airway defects.

KEYWORDS: TRACHEA, ANATOMY; TRACHEOSTOMY

10. Define medical audit. Write short notes on (a) the NCEPOD, and (b) the confidential enquiries into maternal deaths.

Audit

Audit is a system of assessment of performance, also defined as a systematic official scrutiny or a quality check. It involves collection and analysis of data leading to conclusions and recommendations to improve quality of practice or service. In medicine, audit should not interfere with routine clinical practices. Data are usually of the observational or descriptive type, and are collected without resort to standardisation, randomisation, controlling, or blinding. This, together with lack of hypothesis and experiment, is in clear contrast to research and research methods.

(a) NCEPOD

This is the National Confidential Enquiry into Perioperative Deaths. It is an annual audit, since 1988, of all the deaths occurring 0–30 days after any surgical procedure carried out by a surgeon or gynaecologist under general anaesthesia, local anaesthesia or sedation. The enquiry covers almost all hospitals in England, Wales, and Northern Ireland. Apart from collection of data on all the deaths for a general statistic, a sample of cases is selected for detailed questionnaire, data collection, and in-depth analysis. The criteria of selection of each sample vary from year to year, for example "children up to 10 years of age" sample in the 1989 enquiry, or "selective surgical procedures" sample in the 1992 enquiry. A detailed report is published each year highlighting aspects of the quality of care in the perioperative period, patterns of workload, and trends of remediable problems, and recommending standards for organisational and clinical practices.

(b) CEMD

This is the Confidential Enquiries into Maternal Deaths, a triennial statistic of all the deaths of women occurring during pregnancy or within 42 days of its termination. The deaths are from any cause related to the pregnancy or its management, but not from accidental or incidental causes. The enquiry covers all the maternal deaths in the UK (prior to 1984 it covered England, Wales, Scotland, and Northern Ireland separately). The collection and analysis of data of each case report is supervised by the regional obstetric assessors. This is carefully coordinated with the obstetricians, anaesthetists, and pathologists involved, with the help of general practitioners and directors of public health. The national data for the whole of a three-year period are compiled and re-analysed, and a detailed triennial report is then published with descriptive statistics, graphs, and trends of mortality and its

KEYWORDS: AUDIT; NCEPOD; CEMD; MATERNAL DEATHS

causes. Details of individual cases of special interest are also included with the intention of highlighting problems and learning lessons. The CEMD is considered the gold standard, the longest running and the most reputable clinical audit in the world.

KEYWORDS: AUDIT; NCEPOD; CEMD; MATERNAL DEATHS

11. List the indications, contraindications, and complications, of stellate ganglion block.

Indications

- Chronic pain states
  - causalgia
  - reflex sympathetic dystrophy
- Peripheral vascular disease
  - acute vascular disorders, for example inadvertent intra-arterial injection of thiopentone, postembolectomy
  - chronic vasospastic diseases, for example Reynaud's disease

Contraindications

- Anticoagulants and haemorrhagic disorders
- Local infection or neoplasm
- Local anatomical or vascular anomalies
- Patient refusal

Complications

- Systemic toxicity (almost immediate effect if injected into the vertebral arteries)
- Pneumothorax
- Brachial plexus block
- Recurrent laryngeal nerve block (causes temporary hoarseness)
- Phrenic nerve block (causes hemidiaphragmatic paralysis)
- Vagus nerve block (causes tachycardia)
- Cardiac accelerator nerve block (causes bradycardia)
- Subarachnoid injection (if injected into a "dural sleeve")

KEYWORDS: STELLATE GANGLION BLOCK

12. Outline the advantages and disadvantages of performing a transurethral resection of the prostate (TURP) using regional anaesthesia rather than general anaesthesia.

Advantages of regional anaesthesia

- Allows early warning of acute H_2O intoxication (TUR syndrome).
- Reduced blood loss.
- Good postoperative analgesia.
- No mental confusion and easier recovery.
- Avoidance of respiratory failure in patients with chronic obstructive airways disease.
- Avoidance of pulmonary complications in patients with chronic pulmonary disorders.
- Reduced incidence of deep vein thrombosis.

Disadvantages of regional anaesthesia

- Not all patients accept being awake during surgery.
- Patient co-operation is important for success and therefore not suitable if patient is unable to lie still.
- Contraindications exist–absolute and relative:
  - local sepsis
  - disorders of haemostasis
  - fixed cardiac output
  - gross spinal deformities
- Complications may occur:
  - immediate–hypotension, bradycardia, total spinal, intravascular injection of local anaesthetic
  - late–arachnoiditis, meningitis, epidural haematoma, epidural abscess, spinal artery syndrome.

KEYWORDS: TURP; TRANSURETHRAL RESECTION OF PROSTATE

Paper B

1. Outline the causes of immediate postoperative hypoxaemia.

2. Describe the different waves that can be seen in a central venous pressure trace. Give examples of disease that can alter these waves.

3. Draw and label the right first rib. Give a short account of its relations and attachments.

4. Summarise the advantages and disadvantages of total intravenous anaesthesia. What do you understand by "target-controlled infusion"?

5. Write notes on the prophylactic measures that may be used to prevent stress ulcers in patients on the ITU. What are the advantages and disadvantages of these methods?

6. Briefly outline your plan of management for anaesthetising a patient with a permanent pacemaker.

7. What are the warning signs of eclampsia? List the benefits and problems of the available prophylactic anticonvulsant therapies.

8. Design a protocol for the immediate management of anaphylaxis during anaesthesia.

9. What methods are available to measure and reduce intracranial pressure?

10. Briefly describe the possible techniques of anaesthetising the larynx for awake fibreoptic intubation.

11. Describe the immediate management of a 38 year-old hypothermic patient (29°C) presenting in the accident and emergency department.

12. What factors should be considered in the preoperative preparation of a 4 year-old child presenting for correction of a squint?

1. Outline the causes of immediate postoperative hypoxaemia.

The causes of early postoperative hypoxaemia include diffusion hypoxia as a result of nitrous oxide anaesthesia. The commonest categories are listed and discussed below.

* *Hypoventilation*

This commonly arises from upper airway obstruction in the unconscious patient, central respiratory depression which is usually caused by opiates, or respiratory muscle weakness which can result from inadequate reversal of muscle relaxants.

* *Ventilation/perfusion abnormalities*

This arises from prolonged anaesthesia in patients with other systemic diseases such as chronic bronchitis. Abdominal surgery can exacerbate this cause.

* *Increased oxygen consumption*

This can occur in the patient who is cold and is often made worse by shivering.

* *Impaired response to hypoxaemia*

Anaesthesia especially with the volatile anaesthetic agents can impair the normal response to hypoxia and therefore hypoxaemia can occur.

* *Decreased oxygen content*

This can occur after major surgery that has especially been complicated by haemorrhage. A low cardiac output and a low haemoglobin will account for this cause.

For the above reasons, 40% oxygen is routinely given to patients immediately after anaesthesia.

KEYWORDS: POSTOPERATIVE HYPOXAEMIA

2. Describe the different waves that can be seen in a central venous pressure trace. Give examples of disease that can alter these waves.

A typical central venous pressure (CVP) waveform in health would appear like this:

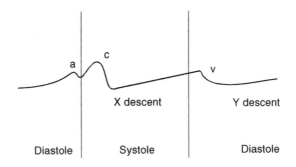

The "a" wave is a positive deflection caused by atrial contraction.

The "c" wave represents the initial bulging of the tricuspid valve into the atrium with the onset of ventricular contraction and the sharp increase in ventricular pressure. The adjacent pulse of the carotid artery also makes a contribution, hence the name "c" wave.

The "x" descent follows as the atrium relaxes and the tricuspid valve is pulled downward during ventricular contraction.

The "v" wave is a positive deflection that occurs as blood accumulates in the vena cavae and right atrium whilst the tricuspid valve is closed.

The "y" descent results from opening of the tricuspid valve and the start of right ventricular filling.

The waves of the CVP trace may alter in disease as follows:

- The "a" wave is absent from CVP traces in patients with atrial fibrillation. This is due to ineffective atrial contraction.
- Large "a" wave amplitude is seen when the atrium contracts against an increased resistance. This occurs in tricuspid stenosis, decreased right ventricular compliance, increased right ventricular pressure from an increased afterload, such as in pulmonary valve stenosis or pulmonary hypertension.
- Giant "a" waves or "cannon" waves occur when the atrium contracts against a closed tricuspid valve. This occurs with cardiac dysrhythmias

KEYWORDS: CENTRAL VENOUS PRESSURE (CVP)

when the atrial and ventricular contractions are not synchronous, such as with nodal or ventricular rhythms or complete heart block.

- Absence of an "x" descent with a large c–v wave is seen in tricuspid regurgitation from valve incompetence. This is caused by pressure in the right atrium rising caused by regurgitation of the blood during ventricular contraction.
- Hypovolaemia may change mean CVP measurement and dampen its trace, but does not specifically alter the shape of its waveforms.

KEYWORDS: CENTRAL VENOUS PRESSURE (CVP)

3. Draw and label the right first rib. Give a short account of its relations and attachments.

The first rib is illustrated below.

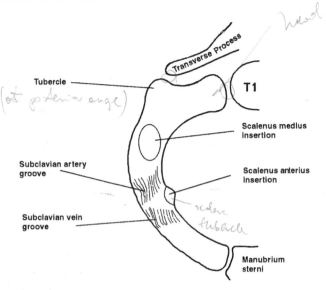

The first rib forms the boundary of the thoracic inlet with the first thoracic vertebra posteriorly and the manubrium sterni anteriorly, and has important neurovascular and musculoskeletal relations. Sibson's fascia or the suprapleural membrane attaches to the inner margin of the first rib. This fibrous layer originates from the transverse process of C7 and spreads over the cervical part of the pleura and lung to provide a protective tent. To the outer margin of the rib attaches serratus anterior and the intercostal muscles of the first space. The head of the rib has a facet which articulates with the body of the first thoracic vertebra (T1). The large tubercle at the posterior angle of the rib articulates with the transverse process of T1. The scalene tubercle provides the insertion for the scalenus anterius tendon. The area of insertion of the scalenus medius is marked in the figure. To the front of the scalene tubercle lies the groove for the subclavian vein, and immediately behind this tubercle is the groove for the subclavian artery. The trunks of the brachial plexus pass between the two areas of insertion of the scalene muscles, just behind and lateral to the subclavian artery.

KEYWORDS: RIB ANATOMY, FIRST

4. Summarise the advantages and disadvantages of total intravenous anaesthesia. What do you understand by "target-controlled infusion"?

Total intravenous anaesthesia

Advantages

- Avoids pollution.
- Avoids the use of N_2O. Diffusion of N_2O to body gaseous spaces may be harmful, for example in ear surgery or in patients with pneumothorax. Prolonged anaesthesia with N_2O also carries a risk of bone marrow depression.
- Does not require anaesthetic machines or vaporisers. May be used in field anaesthesia.
- Less incidence of postoperative nausea and vomiting. This applies to total intravenous anaesthesia with propofol and *not* ketamine or methohexitone!
- Easy and rapid control of induction of anaesthesia and rapid control on the change of depth of anaesthesia during the maintenance period.
- Administration of anaesthesia is independent of airway patency and ventilation. For example, depth of anaesthesia can be maintained during bronchospasm or breath-holding. Another example is the maintenance of anaesthesia during fibreoptic intubation, laryngoscopy, or bronchoscopy with oxygen insufflation or oxygen jet ventilation.
- Suitable for certain conditions such as malignant hyperpyrexia, especially when a vapour-free anaesthetic machine is not available, or in patients with latex allergy where latex material is incorporated in many of the rubber parts of the anaesthetic machine, circuit, and ventilator.

Disadvantages

- Requires repeated injections or reliable infusion devices.
- Unpredictable dose requirement.
- Body movements during surgery in unparalysed patients. Doses that are required to prevent such movements are usually associated with respiratory and cardiovascular depression.
- Risk of awareness in paralysed patients. This is due to the complexity of the pharmacokinetic profile of intravenous anaesthetics with the variability of time constants of distribution and elimination in different individuals.
- Unlike inhalational anaesthetics which can be removed from the body by ventilation, intravenous anaesthetics once injected or infused cannot be removed other than by metabolism or excretion.
- Often more expensive than inhalational anaesthesia.

KEYWORDS: TOTAL INTRAVENOUS ANAESTHESIA (TIVA); TARGET-CONTROLLED INFUSION

27

Target-controlled infusion (TCI)

This is an intravenous infusion system which allows the operator to select the desired target drug concentration in the blood of the patient receiving the infusion. The system, which incorporates a syringe pump and a computerised controller, delivers the infusion at a variable rate determined by an electronic algorithm based on a set of validated pharmacokinetic compartmental-model equations from previous studies with the drug concerned. In anaesthesia TCI was recently introduced with propofol as the intravenous anaesthetic agent.

KEYWORDS: TOTAL INTRAVENOUS ANAESTHESIA (TIVA); TARGET-CONTROLLED INFUSION

5. Write notes on the prophylactic measures that may be used to prevent stress ulcers in patients on the ITU. What are the advantages and disadvantages of these methods?

Feeding

Controversy exists as to how feeding helps to reduce stress ulcers. Intraluminal feeding may act as a buffer or provide nutrients to the mucosal wall and therefore help it to function more effectively as a barrier. Cannot always be used as there may be a contraindication to feeding.

Sucralfate

An aluminium salt of sucrose sulphate that acts as a cytoprotective agent probably by a local action that improves mucosal blood flow. The integrity of the mucosal barrier is maintained without altering pH. It is cheap and has a very low toxicity. May produce hypophosphataemia as the aluminium chelates phosphate in the gut.

Antacids

Often very difficult to titrate the amount of antacid required to produce the desired rise in pH. Stops the antimicrobial action of low gastric pH.

H$_2$-antagonists

More effective at consistently raising gastric pH than antacids. Stops the antimicrobial action of low gastric pH. Relatively expensive. Cimetidine is not commonly used because of its action as a hepatic enzyme inhibitor and its tendency to accumulate if renal function is impaired.

Optimise splanchnic perfusion

Ensuring optimal perfusion pressures and oxygen delivery to the splanchnic bed is very important in the prevention of mucosal injury. Most attempts at monitoring perfusion, such as tonometry, are as yet of unproven value.

KEYWORDS: STRESS ULCERS

6. Briefly outline your plan of management for anaesthetising a patient with a permanent pacemaker.

Preoperative assessment: this includes identification of the primary pathology, the indication for the pacemaker and the pacemaker type and generic code, as shown below (these details may be found in the patient's pacemaker card).

Pacing	Sensing	Response
O	O	O
A	A	I
V	V	T
D	D	D

NB: O = none; A = atrium; V = ventricle; D = dual; T = trigger and I = inhibit.

VVI is the commonest mode. It represents ventricular pacing, ventricular sensing, with inhibition of pacing when a ventricular beat is sensed.

Preoperative assessment also includes a chest X-ray to identify the site of the pacemaker unit and its leads, and an ECG to check the pacing spikes and the intrinsic cardiac rhythm. The heart rate is pacemaker dependent if spikes present before most of the beats.

Intraoperative: preparation in theatre should include ensuring a magnet is available in case a change to VOO pacing is required. This change renders the pacing less susceptible to interference but makes some pacemakers more vulnerable to reprogramming by external stimuli. Resuscitation drugs such as atropine and isoprenaline should be prepared and the defibrillator checked. ECG monitoring is essential perioperatively.

During the operation the risk of microshock/burn must be minimised. It should be remembered that pacemaker leads provide direct access to the electrical current. Arrhythmias may be induced, the pacemaker may be damaged, pacemaker sensing may be triggered with resultant inappropriate inhibition, or the pacemaker may be reprogrammed to a different mode. Diathermy should ideally be avoided, or if necessary bipolar diathermy used. If unipolar diathermy is deemed necessary a minimum duration and intensity may be allowed. The diathermy lead and plate should be positioned away from the chest to ensure the current between the two does not traverse the chest.

Postoperative: the function of the pacemaker should be checked. This should include a 12-lead ECG and if necessary a check at the pacemaker clinic. This is especially important if the anaesthetist suspects that the pacemaker

KEYWORDS: PACEMAKERS

was reprogrammed or showed any significant change in function from its preoperative status. Ideally, the patient's regular pacemaker clinic should be informed of any procedure the patient undergoes involving diathermy.

KEYWORDS: PACEMAKERS

7. What are the warning signs of eclampsia? List the benefits and problems of the available prophylactic anticonvulsant therapies.

Warning signs

Typical warning signs of eclampsia are:

- headache
- nausea
- epigastric or hypochondrial pain
- blurring of vision in a patient with proteinuric gestational hypertension.

However, it should be remembered that eclampsia has been described in patients without the development of these warning signs and even prior to any evidence of proteinuria or gestational hypertension.

Prophylactic anticonvulsant therapies

These can be categorised into three major types:

Benzodiazepines

Benefits
- Effective in treating convulsions. Controversy exists about their role in prophylaxis (see problems).

Problems
- High risk of unconsciousness, pulmonary aspiration and respiratory depression.
- Neonatal hypotonia.

Owing to the high risk of complications, diazepam or other benzodiazepines are no longer recommended for prophylaxis. This has been emphasised in many of the "Confidential Enquiries into Maternal Deaths" reports.

Phenytoin

Benefits
- Little or no effect on the level of consciousness.

Problems
- Variable effectiveness.
- Narrow therapeutic window with its therapeutic dose very close to the toxic dose.
- Zero order kinetics with a fixed rate of metabolism and elimination.
- ATPase stimulator with risk of arrhythmias, hence the need for ECG monitoring during the loading dose.

KEYWORDS: ECLAMPSIA WARNING SIGNS; OBSTETRICS; ANTICONVULSANTS

- Other side effects include pain on injection, hypotension, nausea, vomiting, and nystagmus.
- Requires interval measurements of plasma levels.

Phenytoin is still widely used in the UK and many parts of Europe.

Magnesium sulphate

Benefits
- Probably more effective than phenytoin.
- Little or no effect on the level of consciousness.

Problems
- Unknown mechanism of action and a potential for drug interaction.
- Requires measurements of plasma levels.
- Reduces the liberation of acetylcholine at the neuromuscular junction, and depresses the excitability of the endplate, and the muscle membrane. Hence, the increased sensitivity to both depolarising and non-depolarising muscle relaxants.
- Hypotonia in mother and newborn.

Universally used in North America, widely used in Australia and South Africa, and now increasingly used in the UK.

KEYWORDS: ECLAMPSIA WARNING SIGNS; OBSTETRICS; ANTICONVULSANTS

8. Design a protocol for the immediate management of anaphylaxis during anaesthesia.

Anaphylaxis should be suspected when sudden hypotension, tachycardia, bronchospasm, and urticaria occur soon after the administration of a drug.

Action

- Stop the suspected drug.
- Call for help.
- Stop surgery if appropriate.
- Give oxygen 100%.
- Commence CPR if no output.
- Elevate legs.
- Secure large intravenous cannula.
- Adrenaline is the drug of choice. Aim for 100 micrograms/minute for an average adult. Use 1:10 000 solution and give 1 ml every minute intravenously and titrate according to the response.
- Start intravenous fluid, colloid 10–20 ml/kg.
- Establish continuous ECG monitoring. This should already be in place as an essential monitor.
- Establish pulse oximetry and capnography if not already in place.
- If bronchospasm persists consider one or more of the following bronchodilators; sulbutamol 2.5–5 mg nebulised or 250 micrograms intravenously or aminophylline 250 mg intravenously.
- Consider insertion of a central venous line.

Further measures

- Consider IPPV.
- Consider insertion of arterial line and taking an arterial sample for blood gas and acid-base analysis.
- Consider antihistamine for flushing and urticaria.
- Steroids are controversial and not conclusive.
- Take venous blood samples as soon as is possible for FBC, APTT, PT and fibrinogen. Repeat samples 6-hourly for 12–24 hours to exclude haemolysis, clotting derangements, and disseminated intravascular coagulopathy.
- Take venous blood samples for allergy studies. Collect in EDTA tube as soon as possible and send to the laboratory to spin off the plasma and store at − 20°C. Repeat at 3, 6 and 24 hours.

KEYWORDS: ANAPHYLAXIS

9. What methods are available to measure and reduce intracranial pressure?

Intracranial pressure is measured to give an indication of cerebral perfusion pressure, to assess the possibility of "coning", in the monitoring of neurological status in ITU and in the management of cerebral oedema and hydrocephalus. Normal intracranial pressure is < 10 mmHg and a pressure of > 20 mmHg should be a cause for concern.

The methods of measuring intracranial pressure are listed below:

- Intraventricular catheter connected to a transducer–accurate but infection risk
- Subdural devices
  - bolt (Richmond screw)
  - catheter
- Extradural devices
  - bolt
  - Gaeltec–transducer at catheter tip
  - Ladd–fibreoptic system with mirrors

Methods to reduce intracranial pressure include those listed below:

- Surgical removal of an intracranial lesion
- Hyperventilation to a Pa_{CO_2} of 4.5 kPa
- Drainage of CSF via an intraventricular catheter
- 20% mannitol
- Dexamethasone
- Intravenous induction agents except ketamine
- 15 degree head up tilt–promotes venous drainage
- Neutral head and neck position with unobstructed venous outflow

KEYWORDS: INTRACRANIAL PRESSURE

10. Briefly describe the possible techniques of anaesthetising the larynx for awake fibreoptic intubation.

There are 3 different techniques.

1. *Transtracheal injection* of local anaesthetic. Draw 3 ml of lignocaine 4% in a 5 ml syringe and attach to a 22 G hypodermic needle. Wipe the area of the cricothyroid membrane with antiseptic. Feel the gap between the thyroid and cricoid cartilages and insert the needle in the mid-line and perpendicular to the skin. A sudden give way (pop) at a depth of 1–2 cm with aspiration of air confirms the placement of the needle in the trachea. Inject and pull the needle out rapidly as this is followed immediately by a violent cough. The cough is useful in spreading the local anaesthetic in the trachea and up to the larynx.

2. *Superior laryngeal nerve block.* Draw 5 ml of lignocaine 1% in a 5 ml syringe. Clean with antiseptic the skin overlaying the hyoid bone on each side of the neck. Start on one side. Insert a 22 G needle perpendicular to the skin and 0.5 cm caudad to the cornu of the hyoid bone. Advance 0.5–1 cm, aspirate to exclude intravascular placement of the needle, and infiltrate 2.5 ml. Repeat the same technique on the other side injecting the other 2.5 ml.

3. *Topical anaesthesia* or "spray as you go" technique. A maximum of 4 ml anhydrous lignocaine 4% solution or 10 doses from the 10% lignocaine spray pump may be used to spray the larynx. Alternatively, 2–4 ml of 4% lignocaine may be injected through the suction channel of the fibrescope as soon as the glottis comes to view and before entering the larynx.

KEYWORDS: LARYNX; FIBREOPTIC INTUBATION

11. Describe the immediate management of a 38-year-old hypothermic patient (29°C) presenting in the accident and emergency department.

This is a medical emergency. The patient is in severe hypothermia and is likely to be unconscious. The basic rules of resuscitation apply, so airway, breathing, and circulation are a priority, and cardiopulmonary resuscitation should be started without delay if indicated. The patient then needs to be slowly warmed whilst any metabolic abnormalities are corrected and any cardiac dysrhythmias treated. There should also be a search for any underlying cause.

- *Airway* – Unless there is a clear history of no trauma to the head and neck area, a hard collar should be applied until cervical spine injury has been excluded. With this conscious level it is highly likely that the patient's protective airway reflexes are obtunded and so he or she should be intubated with a cuffed endotracheal tube. After preoxygenation, a greatly reduced dose of induction agent should be given and cricoid pressure applied. Suxamethonium should then be given and the trachea intubated.

- *Breathing* – Breathing should be assisted until it is clear that the patient's own breathing is adequate. Arterial blood gases should be taken, but their interpretation should allow correction for the patient's body temperature.

- *Circulation* – The patient should have blood pressure and ECG monitored. Hypotension should initially be treated with warmed fluids. If this proves unsuccessful, it may be necessary to start inotropes. The presence of arrhythmias such as asystole and ventricular fibrillation should be watched for and treated according to resuscitation protocol.

- *Warming* – The patient should be slowly but actively warmed (1 degree Celsius per hour) by using warming blankets, a warm room and warmed intravenous fluids. A heat and moisture exchanger should be included in the breathing system. Techniques such as peritoneal lavage and haemofiltration are suggested but are rarely used to rewarm patients in these circumstances.

- *Metabolic disturbances* are variable. The patient may have either a metabolic acidosis or alkalosis. In general neither of these would be treated unless they were thought to be severely compromising the patient cardiovascularly. Hypoglycaemia is common and should be actively looked for and managed.

KEYWORDS: HYPOTHERMIA

12. What factors should be considered in the pre-operative preparation of a 4 year-old child presenting for correction of a squint?

Considerations for squint correction

- Possible association with other conditions, for example Cruzon's and Apert's syndromes or malignant hyperthermia.
- Need for psychological preparation. Addressing and allaying parental concerns are important in establishing the trust and confidence of the child. Contact between the child and anaesthetist before anaesthesia positively affects the quality of induction and overall experience of the child.
- Need for pharmacological premedication.
- Parental presence at induction.
- Suitability of procedure and child for day-case surgery. Several factors have allowed day-case squint correction to be performed with a very low incidence of postoperative morbidity–availability of EMLA cream, propofol, and the reinforced laryngeal mask airway which alleviates the need for endotracheal intubation and muscle relaxation. Suitability for day surgery depends on ASA status (1 or 2), home, and social circumstances. The preoperative preparation should include the following:
  - a written and verbal explanation to the parents about the surgical procedure, preparations to be made, the postoperative course and their involvement in the care of the child;
  - an explanation to the child appropriate to child's ability to understand;
  - a pre-admission programme using play simulation, photographs, videos etc;
  - information about fasting requirements.
- Possible intraoperative problems in relation to this operation. Oculocardiac reflex–elicited by surgeon when applying traction to the extraocular muscles especially the medial rectus and lateral rectus. Usually causes bradycardia but occasionally other arrhythmias. Prophylactic measures such as intravenous atropine 20 micrograms/kg or glycopyrrolate 10 micrograms/kg are required at induction.

KEYWORDS: CHILDREN, SQUINT

Paper C

1. A 45-year-old man has been rescued with extensive burns from a house fire. Outline your management of the problems that may be encountered in the first 24 hours.

2. Write short notes on the causes, diagnosis, and treatment of a pneumothorax occurring during anaesthesia.

3. Write a short essay on cystic fibrosis with special reference to anaesthesia.

4. Give details of the current clinical uses of magnesium.

5. Outline the problems of anaesthesia for a 20 year-old heroin addict requiring drainage of an arm abscess.

6. Draw a labelled diagram of the antecubital fossa. Outline the management of accidental intra-arterial injection of thiopentone in the upper limb.

7. A patient requires intubation and has four capped incisor teeth. What would you tell him preoperatively? During a difficult intubation two caps are subsequently knocked out. What would you do?

8. Describe how you would diagnose and manage a patient with massive pulmonary embolism.

9. Outline the anaesthetic techniques available for a bronchoscopy.

10. Define the acute respiratory distress syndrome, and describe what methods can be used to improve oxygenation in this condition.

11. Briefly describe the physical principles involved in pulse oximetry.

12. Discuss the problems of anaesthesia for a patient who is to be placed in the prone position.

1. A 45 year-old man has been rescued with extensive burns from a house fire. Outline your management of the problems that may be encountered in the first 24 hours.

Immediate

The immediate problems from a severe burn are:
- Hypovolaemia from loss of plasma.
- Airway oedema and respiratory complications from inhalation of poisonous or hot gases.
- Difficulty with tracheal intubation in the presence of facial or airway burns.
- Pain.
- Metabolic effects from a highly catabolic state.
- Infection risks from loss of skin barrier, dead tissue, and immunodeficiency.

As many of the above are life-threatening complications, it is appropriate that experienced personnel are involved in the patient's management from the outset. Following resuscitation and stabilisation, arrangements must be made to transfer him to a specialist burns unit.

Management

Management includes:
(1) *Initial treatment*
  - Assessment of airway, breathing, circulation, and conscious level.
  - 100% oxygen via a tight-fitting face mask connected to an anaesthetic machine.
  - Intubation and ventilation if unconscious or if evidence of smoke inhalation. Intubation can prove to be difficult or even impossible by conventional methods. Suxamethonium is considered safe in the first 24 hours following a burn injury.
  - Intravenous access–may be difficult.
  - Blood for FBC, U&Es, cross-match, ABGs, and carboxyhaemoglobin.
  - Secondary survey to exclude other injuries he may have sustained in an attempt to escape.
  - Assessment of the extent of burn (rule of nine)–depth, surface area.
  - Intravenous opioid analgesia.
  - Urinary catheter.
  - Nasogastric tube (to prevent acute dilatation of the stomach).

KEYWORDS: BURNS

(2) *Fluid replacement*
   - Various formulae; colloid/crystalloid (colloid favoured in the UK).
   - Type and amount depend on pulse, BP, urine, haematocrit, CVP.
   - Frequent reassessments crucial to guide therapy.

(3) *Inhalational injury*

Indicators: fire in an enclosed space; stridor/wheeze; burns to the head and neck and/or circumferential burns; coughing of soot-stained sputum; burnt nasal hair and eyebrows; impaired consciousness. Fibreoptic bronchoscopy is useful to assess the extent and severity of the airway and lung injury. Direct thermal injury, toxic gases and smoke inhalation cause:

   - supraglottic oedema
   - damage to distal airways and lung parenchyma
   - carbon monoxide poisoning: suspect clinically and confirm by co-oximetry.

Treatment: administer 100% oxygen which reduces the half-life of carboxyhaemoglobin from 4 hours to < 1 hour; intubate and ventilate if unconscious; hyperbaric oxygen therapy for severe cases (COHb level > 40%).

   - Cyanide poisoning–suspect if metabolic acidosis, high blood lactate; treatment–amyl nitrite, sodium thiosulphate.

(4) *Hypothermia*–nurse in warm environment.

(5) *Nutrition*–early enteral feeding because of high catabolic state.

(6) *Stress ulcer prophylaxis.*

(7) *Definitive treatment*
   - Infection–isolation, topical antibiotics, tetanus toxoid.
   - Surgery–escharotomy, dressing, early grafts.

KEYWORDS: BURNS

2. Write short notes on the causes, diagnosis, and treatment of a pneumothorax occurring during anaesthesia.

Causes

- *Injury by needle*: injuries to pleura and lungs with needles such as during insertion of a central venous cannula, supraclavicular brachial plexus block, intercostal nerve block or intrapleural block and rarely thoracic epidural block.
- *Anaesthetic machine*: barotrauma, as a result of pressure transmitted from the gas supply, cylinders or oxygen flush system; also high inflation pressures during IPPV, or accidental occlusion of expiratory limb or a pressure relief valve in the patient's circuit.
- *Trauma to the airway*: injuries to the larynx, trachea, and carina during instrumentation of the airway, for example during induction of anaesthesia and especially in a difficult intubation situation.
- *Patient factors*: some patients are more prone to developing a pneumothorax. Asthmatic patients and patients with chronic obstructive airway diseases require high inflation pressures during IPPV and have high alveolar trapping volumes; patients with congenital lung bullae and patients with previous trauma to the chest may develop pneumothorax after IPPV.
- *Surgical factors*: some surgical procedures such as nephrectomy, operations on the thoracic spine, operations on the larynx, and obviously cardiac and thoracic operations, are associated with high risk of pneumothorax.

Diagnosis

- Diminished air entry on the affected side.
- Resonance to percussion on the affected side.
- Diminished expansion of the affected side.
- Diminished auscultation sounds on the affected side.
- Shift of trachea, only if tension pneumothorax, to the opposite side.
- Surgical emphysema, felt as crepitus under the skin and soft tissues when palpated against bone such as a clavicle, is characteristic of trauma-related pneumothorax with injuries to the chest wall. It may also occur with tension pneumothorax.
- High airway ventilatory pressures.
- Drop in Sao_2 is a late sign especially during anaesthesia with Fio_2 of ≥ 0.3.
- Hypotension, especially in tension pneumothorax, from increased intrathoracic pressure and reduced venous return.
- Chest X-ray will confirm the diagnosis but this should not delay treatment if tension pneumothorax is suspected.

KEYWORDS: PNEUMOTHORAX

Treatment

- Insertion of a chest drain in the 4th–5th intercostal space at the mid-axillary line, with connection to an underwater seal drainage.
- In the case of tension pneumothorax, immediate action is necessary. Drainage of the air may be achieved quickly by inserting a wide bore needle in the 2nd intercostal space at the mid-clavicular line.

KEYWORDS: PNEUMOTHORAX

3. Write a short essay on cystic fibrosis with special reference to anaesthesia.

Cystic fibrosis or mucoviscidosis is an inherited autosomal recessive disorder of the exocrine glands. The cells which are relatively impermeable to electrolytes secrete thick electrolyte-rich viscid mucus which blocks and damages the affected glands. This also causes abnormal elevation of sweat salts, and increased organic and enzymatic constituents of intestinal secretions. The glands most affected are those in the pancreas and respiratory system. Salivary and sweat glands are also affected.

Patients commonly present as infants or children and many die from terminal respiratory failure early in their adulthood. As neonates they may present with meconium ileus. Later, as children and in early adulthood, they present with repeated chest infections complicated by bronchiectasis and emphysema. Poor nutritional status due to pancreatic insufficiency, steatorrhoea, and distal intestinal obstruction syndrome is another recognised feature of the disease. Associated medical conditions with this disorder are overactivity of the autonomic nervous system and diabetes.

Prophylactic antibiotics should be considered to reduce chest infections in these patients. This is especially true for perioperative chest infections. Bronchodilators and mucolytic agents are commonly used to reduce any obstructive elements and help liquefy the retained thick tenacious mucus. Physiotherapy such as postural drainage and breathing exercises plays an important role in dislodging the secretions and improving pulmonary functions.

Selected patients are considered for lung or heart–lung transplantation surgery.

KEYWORDS: CYSTIC FIBROSIS

4. Give details of the current clinical uses of magnesium.

Magnesium is currently used in a variety of clinical situations:

- To treat *hypomagnesaemia*. This is a common problem on the intensive care unit and it has been shown that correction of abnormally low magnesium levels helps in the process of ventilatory weaning.
- In the management of *tachyarrhythmias*. Magnesium is a co-factor for $Na^+-K^+ATPase$. With hypomagnesaemia, intracellular potassium will be depleted. Magnesium may also have some intrinsic antiarrhythmic action and is particularly useful in the treatment of torsade des pointes, multifocal atrial tachycardia and the ventricular arrhythmia seen with digitalis intoxication.
- In the treatment of *eclampsia*. Throughout a large part of the western world, magnesium is now well established as the first-line treatment of eclampsia. It is currently gaining in popularity in the UK. Magnesium antagonises calcium at membrane channels and reduces cerebral vasospasm. It produces a similar effect on the systemic vasculature and along with its inhibitory action on catecholamine release, magnesium has a mild antihypertensive action. Magnesium is also a tocolytic and therefore improves uterine blood flow. It is sometimes given to obtund the hypertensive response to intubation in eclampsia. Investigations into the role of magnesium in the prophylaxis of eclampsia have failed to show any benefit.
- As a treatment for *constipation*. Magnesium is now used less for this condition, as bulking agents such as Fybogel, and suppositories and enemas are becoming more widely used.
- Possibly in the management of patients following *myocardial infarction*. The LIMIT-II study showed an improvement in survival postinfarction in the group given magnesium. This was not confirmed by a larger study and, because of side effects, magnesium is currently not recommended in the management of acute myocardial infarction.
- In the management of *severe asthma*. Magnesium has been used in the treatment of severe refractory asthma. It is thought to block calcium channels and to inhibit parasympathetic acetylcholine release.
- *Hypocalcaemia*. Hypomagnesaemia may exacerbate hypocalcaemia by inhibiting the release and action of parathyroid hormone.
- *Tetanus*. Magnesium has been used as an adjunct to sedation in the treatment of tetanus.

KEYWORDS: MAGNESIUM THERAPY

5. Outline the problems of anaesthesia for a 20 year-old heroin addict requiring drainage of an arm abscess.

This problem needs to be assessed firstly from the point of view of the addiction:

- Heroin addicts can be unreliable when giving a clinical history and may not give accurate histories of operations and previous medical illnesses.
- Venous access which is mandatory prior to anaesthesia can be impossible and occasionally surgical cut-down is necessary.
- Acute intoxication may be apparent and the co-operation of the patient may be difficult.
- Drug withdrawal can occur in hospital and must be managed by appropriate professionals including social workers and psychiatrists.
- Associated addictions can occur which may have physical consequences for the patient. These include alcohol and tobacco abuse; when these patients are examined care must be taken to ensure that associated diseases such as cardiomyopathy do not exist.
- Intercurrent infections can exist, especially septicaemia and endocarditis.
- Associated infections can influence the anaesthetist in the management of this case. There is an increased risk of hepatitis and HIV infections and it is the duty of the anaesthetist to prevent personnel, theatre staff, and equipment transmission of these infections. Universal sterility precautions must be undertaken.
- Thrombosis and embolism are a greater risk in this patient.
- Multisystem investigations are needed, as conditions such as thrombocytopenia can occur in this group of patients and may preclude regional anaesthesia.
- Enzyme induction may influence anaesthetic requirements in general anaesthesia.
- Postoperative analgesia is often difficult to manage.

Secondly the type of anaesthesia needs to be considered. This operation can be performed under regional anaesthesia with a brachial plexus block. This, whilst having potential complications such as pneumothorax may be the best technique if there is no infection locally or clotting problems. General anaesthesia may be chosen and in an emergency would necessitate a "rapid sequence induction" technique.

KEYWORDS: DRUG ADDICTION; HEROIN ADDICTION; ARM ABSCESS

6. Draw a labelled diagram of the antecubital fossa. Outline the management of accidental intra-arterial injection of thiopentone in the upper limb.

Antecubital fossa

The antecubital fossa is drawn below:

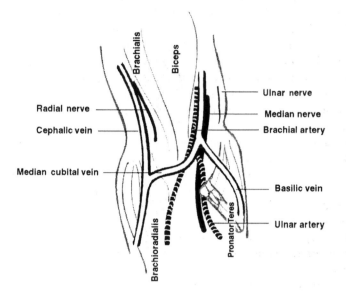

Management of intra-arterial injection of thiopentone

Intra-arterial injection causes intense pain and may cause distal blistering, oedema, and gangrene attributed to crystallisation of thiopentone within arterioles and capillaries, with local noradrenaline release and vasospasm.

- Leave the cannula/needle in the artery and inject the following:
  - saline, to dilute the drug;
  - vasodilators, for example, papaverine 40 mg or phentolamine 2–5 mg, to reduce arterial spasm;
  - procaine 50–100 mg, to reduce pain and produce vasodilatation;
  - heparin, to reduce subsequent thrombosis.
- Brachial plexus block or a stellate ganglion block (before heparinisation) can be considered as they help encourage vasodilatation from sympathetic blockade.
- Postpone surgery.

KEYWORDS: ANTECUBITAL FOSSA ANATOMY; INTRA-ARTERIAL THIOPENTONE

7. A patient requires intubation and has four capped incisor teeth. What would you tell him preoperatively? During a difficult intubation two caps are subsequently knocked out. What would you do?

Preoperatively an explanation of the anaesthetic is needed. The patient should be told that, in general, caps are more fragile than normal, healthy teeth, and that the main reason for asking where the caps are is to allow one to avoid damaging them. It should be stated that, because of their more fragile nature, damage to caps does sometimes occur, although this is rare.

It may be appropriate to use a gumshield during intubation. It may be local policy to get the patient to sign an anaesthetic consent form in the knowledge that capped teeth are at risk.

In the unfortunate event of accidental removal of two capped teeth, the immediate action should be to retrieve the teeth once the airway is secured, or even before if aspiration of one of the caps is likely. The capped teeth should be kept in a safe place. The anaesthetic consultant responsible for the list should be informed. At the end of a short procedure, with the patient awake, extubated, and in control of the airway, it is sometimes possible to insert the teeth successfully back into the gum if some natural tooth and root has also been removed. This, however, is rarely the case.

The whole event should be recorded in detail in the notes. The patient should be visited postoperatively and a full explanation given, including telling the patient that it was a difficult intubation. Local policy should be consulted with regard to the Trust offering to pay for new caps, and the patient should be referred to a dentist.

KEYWORDS: TEETH

8. Describe how you would diagnose and manage a patient with massive pulmonary embolism.

Diagnosis

Relevant history, examination, and investigations should be made with special attention to the points below:

- *Risk factors* include heart failure, cancer, hip fractures, prolonged bed rest, obesity, oestrogen therapy, age over 65 years, antithrombin III deficiency.
- *Symptoms* include sudden onset of dyspnoea, chest pain (substernal or pleuritic), and possibly haemoptysis if pulmonary infarction ensues.
- *Physical signs* include tachypnoea, cyanosis, tachycardia, systemic hypotension, raised CVP. The rise in pulmonary artery pressure may be associated with splitting of the second heart sound and a loud pulmonary component, right ventricular heave and a gallop rhythm. There may be clinical evidence of deep vein thrombosis and a slight fever.
- *ECG*: sinus tachycardia and signs of right ventricular strain are common findings. P pulmonale, right bundle branch block and atrial arrhythmias may also be seen. The classic pattern of S_1,Q_3,T_3 is unusual.
- *CXR* may show large pulmonary arteries, pulmonary oligaemia, pleural effusion, raised hemidiaphragm.
- *Arterial blood gases* show hypoxaemia, metabolic and respiratory acidosis.

Ventilation/perfusion isotope scanning and pulmonary angiography confirm the diagnosis but often clinical judgement must be relied upon in patients with massive pulmonary embolism.

Management

- *Resuscitation*: includes oxygenation and maintenance of the airway, mechanical ventilation, expansion of circulating volume, and inotropic support to maintain right ventricular perfusion.
- *Definitive treatment*: directed towards preventing further thrombus formation and proximal embolisation:
  - thrombolytic therapy such as streptokinase 250 000 units i.v. over 30 minutes, followed by infusion of 100 000 units/h for 24 h; streptokinase is pyrogenic, antigenic, and poses a significant haemorrhagic risk;
  - pulmonary embolectomy may be indicated in a profoundly shocked patient when streptokinase is contraindicated or fails.

KEYWORDS: PULMONARY EMBOLISM

9. Outline the anaesthetic techniques available for a bronchoscopy.

Bronchoscopy can be performed either as a diagnostic or a therapeutic procedure, with the use of either general or regional anaesthesia.

Flexible bronchoscopy is often performed as a diagnostic procedure by chest physicians using local anaesthesia with or without sedation. It is also undertaken as a therapeutic procedure in intensive care unit patients through a tracheal or tracheostomy tube to aspirate sputum plugs. The airway is anaesthetised by direct topical application of non-toxic doses of local anaesthetics. Cricothyroid puncture is occasionally used to anaesthetise the mucosa beneath the level of the vocal cords. If the larynx is anaesthetised, a patient who is vomiting may aspirate gastric contents, and all patients should therefore be routinely fasted before the procedure.

Rigid bronchoscopy is performed under general anaesthesia. Four techniques are used:

(1) spontaneous respiration through the bronchoscope;
(2) apnoeic oxygenation;
(3) intermittent positive pressure ventilation using the Venturi principle;
(4) high frequency ventilation techniques.

In adults the most common technique is the third one, utilising the Venturi principle. Following induction of anaesthesia, the patient is paralysed with a short-acting muscle relaxant, such as suxamethonium. The bronchoscope is inserted and 100% oxygen insufflated with the Sander's injector device which works using the Venturi principle. This technique has risks associated with it and the main ones are awareness, pneumothorax, and the dispersal of blood (and, if relevant, a foreign body) deep into the lungs.

KEYWORDS: BRONCHOSCOPY

10. Define the acute respiratory distress syndrome, and describe what methods can be used to improve oxygenation in this condition.

The acute respiratory distress syndrome (ARDS) is defined as a clinical condition in which the patient has hypoxia, poorly compliant lungs, and high airway pressures. This is ascertained with characteristic chest X-ray findings of diffuse pulmonary infiltrates combined with a normal or low pulmonary artery wedge pressure. There is an underlying pathology from a recognised list that leads to ARDS. The most common causes are trauma and sepsis.

The following methods have been used to improve oxygenation:

- *Raising inspired oxygen concentration (FiO$_2$).* It is desirable to keep the FiO$_2$ below 60%. This is often not possible and the patient may require 100% FiO$_2$
- *Ventilation with PEEP.* The patient is ventilated often with up to 15 cm H$_2$O of PEEP. High airway pressures are often encountered and the patient is at risk of barotrauma.
- *Reverse I:E ratio.* Allowing a longer time in the inspiratory phase of the respiratory cycle often provides enough time for more efficient ventilation of the relatively stiff lung.
- *Pressure controlled ventilation.* With this technique the lungs are inflated to a pre-set pressure. The tidal volume is therefore determined by the compliance of the lung. The upper pressure limit can be increased to recruit previously collapsed sections of lung and maximise the amount of lung available for ventilation. It is often necessary to paralyse patients in addition to their sedation to perform adequate pressure-controlled ventilation.
- *Prone position.* Postural change has often been observed to temporarily improve oxygenation in ARDS. This is probably due to a favourable *V:Q* mismatch. Prone ventilation is, however, not without risk, and meticulous attention to airway management must be observed.
- *Extracorporeal membrane oxygenation (ECMO).* Although ECMO has always seemed to be a good idea in ARDS, it has not been found to be of value in improving outcome in adults.
- *Nitric oxide (nebulised prostacycline)*
- *Permissive hypereapnia*
- *Liquid ventilation*
- *IVOX*

KEYWORDS: ACUTE RESPIRATORY DISTRESS SYNDROME (ARDS)

11. Briefly describe the physical principles involved in pulse oximetry.

Oximetry utilises the different absorption coefficients of different wavelengths of light by oxyhaemoglobin (oxy-Hb) and reduced-haemoglobin (reduced-Hb) to measure oxygen saturation, as in the figure below.

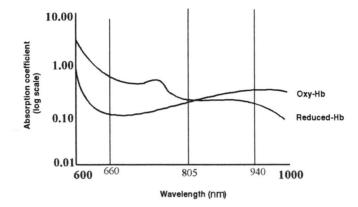

At 660 nm wavelength (red light) reduced-Hb exhibits absorption approximately 10 times that of oxy-Hb while at 940 nm wavelength (near infrared light) oxy-Hb exhibits the higher absorption. At 805 nm wavelength both reduced-Hb and oxy-Hb have similar absorption coefficients. Pulse oximetry operates with two alternating light-emitting diodes and one sensing photodiode placed on opposite sides of a digit or any other suitable part of the body. It uses the isolation and processing of the pulsatile part of the signal of light absorption to verify the arterial component of oxygen saturation, as in the figure below.

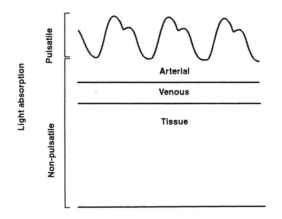

The electronic algorithm used in the substantial sophisticated signal

KEYWORDS: PULSE OXIMETRY

processing is simplified by the equation:

$$X = (P660/P940)/(NP660/NP940)$$

where X is the arterial oxygen saturation, P is the pulsatile component of the absorption coefficient, and NP is the non-pulsatile component of the coefficient.

KEYWORDS: PULSE OXIMETRY

12. Discuss the problems of anaesthesia for a patient who is to be placed in the prone position.

The positioning of a patient for surgery is critical for safe outcome, as damage to limbs, joints, pressure areas and nerves may occur unless care is taken. Proper positioning means that the patient should be securely placed on the operating table, all potential pressure areas padded, intravenous lines and catheter free flowing and accessible, endotracheal tube in proper position, ventilation and circulation uninterrupted, and general patient comfort and safety maintained for the duration of the surgery.

Specific concerns associated with the prone position include:

- Tracheal tubes and intravenous lines may be displaced during movement.
- Access to endotracheal tube is difficult; possibility of kinking and accidental extubation in this position.
- Anteroposterior (A-P) chest expansion is reduced.
- Diaphragmatic excursion can be restricted when support of the shoulders and pelvis is incorrect.
- Venous return may also be impeded if the abdomen is compressed.
- Brachial plexus becomes stretched if the arms are abducted more than 90 degrees.
- The neck should be kept in the neutral position during patient transfer or positioning on the table. It is important to minimise cervical injury (bony or neurological).
- Eyes are vulnerable to injury: corneal abrasions and direct compression of the globe can occur. The retinal artery can become compressed by external pressure, resulting in retinal ischaemia and blindness. This can be prevented by padding around the orbit. Taping the eyes shut and use of eye lubricants reduce the incidence of corneal abrasions and prevent corneal drying.
- Skin breakdown can occur from incorrect positioning. Padding of all pressure points, including the face, arms, knees, hips, ankles, breasts and genitalia, is needed in this position. The patient should also be free from pressure by ECG electrodes, wires, and tubing.
- Resuscitation is difficult in the prone position.

KEYWORDS: PRONE POSITION

Paper D

1. Summarise the ways in which the function of the diaphragm may be affected during general or local anaesthesia.

2. Outline the problems associated with anaesthetising a patient with rheumatoid arthritis.

3. What factors can affect brain damage after a head injury? Explain the Glasgow Coma Scale.

4. Outline the physiological changes that occur during laparoscopy.

5. List, with examples when appropriate, the possible causes of air embolism during surgery, and the methods of diagnosis and treatment.

6. Describe the physiological regulation of cerebral blood flow. Outline how this may be influenced by anaesthesia.

7. Briefly describe the use of filters in (a) blood transfusion, (b) epidural infusions, and (c) breathing systems.

8. Briefly list factors involved in the pathophysiology of septic shock resulting from Gram negative bacterial infections.

9. Outline the preoperative assessment of a patient who requires a partial thyroidectomy. What early complications may result from this operation?

10. Write a short account on the normal distribution curve.

11. Summarise the problems relating to perioperative management of HIV positive patients.

12. Which patient groups are at risk from extravasation injury? How would you manage a case of severe extravasation of thiopentone in the dorsum of a patient's hand.

1. Summarise the ways in which the function of the diaphragm may be affected during general or local anaesthesia.

The diaphragm may be affected in the following ways.

Mechanical

Splinting of the diaphragm by abdominal viscera increases when the supine or lateral positions are adopted from the erect position. This is particularly significant in obese or pregnant patients. The use of a nephrectomy table bridge, or breaking (angling) the table will further compromise the function of the diaphragm. The prone position is associated with further splinting of the diaphragm if the abdomen is not free from the pressure of the operating table. Surgical retractors and abdominal packs obviously limit the movements of the diaphragm. Inflation of the abdomen with CO_2, such as during a laparoscopic procedure, also causes mechanical splinting of the diaphragm.

Pharmacological

Intravenous and inhalational anaesthetics are known to cause weakness of the diaphragm muscle, especially at deep planes of anaesthesia. Depolarising and non-depolarising muscle relaxants paralyse the diaphragm. Local application of aminoglycoside antibiotics, such as in peritoneal lavage, is known to potentiate the effects of non-depolarising muscle relaxants.

Neurological

Paralysis of the phrenic nerve is possible during interscalene or supraclavicular brachial plexus block (for this reason and also because of the risk of pneumothorax, bilateral blocks should not be attempted), local anaesthetic infiltration during the insertion of internal jugular central line, and high spinal or epidural anaesthesia reaching C5 (the phrenic nerve which provides its motor supply originates from C3–5).

KEYWORDS: DIAPHRAGM FUNCTION

2. Outline the problems associated with anaesthetising a patient with rheumatoid arthritis.

Patients with rheumatoid arthritis can present with a number of complex problems arising as a result of the following:

Articular consequences of the disease

- Presence of deformities may compromise positioning during surgery as well as affect access for regional techniques or venous cannulation.
- Rheumatoid involvement of the head and neck may predispose to difficult airway management during anaesthesia:
  - cervical spine–instability, anterior subluxation at axial level, fixed flexion deformities make conventional laryngoscopy difficult, if not impossible;
  - temporomandibular joint–disease produces limitation of mouth opening;
  - cricoarytenoid joints–bilateral fixation can cause airway obstruction.

Systemic consequences of the disease

- *Heart*–pericarditis and effusion, myocarditis, granulomatous disease affecting conduction pathways and heart valves.
- *Lungs*–pleural effusion, interstitial lung fibrosis, nodules, Caplan's syndrome in coal miners, restrictive lung defect.
- *Blood*–normocytic, normo- or hypochromic anaemia, Felty's syndrome with hypersplenism.
- *Kidneys*–function impaired from interstitial nephritis, amyloidosis, drugs.
- *Eyes*–uveiitis, Sjögren's syndrome.
- *Nerves*–mononeuritis, peripheral neuropathy.

Adverse effects of concomitant drug therapy

- *NSAIDs*–deterioration in renal function.
- *Gold*–nephrotic syndrome, immune thrombocytopenia, hepatitis, pneumonitis.
- *Penicillamine*–proteinuria, SLE.
- *Corticosteroids*–cushingoid features.
- *Methotrexate*–gastrointestinal side effects, bone marrow suppression.
- *Cyclosporin*–nephrotoxicity.

KEYWORDS: RHEUMATOID ARTHRITIS

3. What factors can affect brain damage after a head injury? Explain the Glasgow Coma Scale.

The causes can be divided into primary and secondary. Primary damage occurs at the time of the injury. Secondary brain damage occurs at a variable time after the initial insult and is the result of a decrease in cerebral perfusion and oxygenation. The causes of secondary brain damage are as follows:

- Hypoxaemia
- Hypercapnia
- Increased cerebral venous pressure
  - coughing
  - vomiting
  - straining
- Infection
- Hypotension.

The Glasgow Coma Scale (GCS) is a universal system of neurological assessment. Localising signs and pupillary reaction are also noted on the scale. Neurological progress can be assessed by changes in the GCS score. A score of < 8 is serious and is often an indication for tracheal intubation. The scale is as below:

- Best motor response
  - obeys commands   6
  - withdraws from painful stimuli   5
  - localises to painful stimuli   4
  - flexes to painful stimuli   3
  - extends to painful stimuli   2
  - no response   1

- Best verbal response
  - orientated   5
  - confused speech   4
  - inappropriate words   3
  - incomprehensible sounds   2
  - none   1

- Eye opening response
  - spontaneously   4
  - to speech   3
  - to pain   2
  - none   1

KEYWORDS: HEAD INJURY; GLASGOW COMA SCALE; BRAIN DAMAGE; COMA

The GCS is a reliable way of communicating the severity of a head injury to another medical team not involved with the patient.

KEYWORDS: HEAD INJURY; GLASGOW COMA SCALE; BRAIN DAMAGE; COMA

4. Outline the physiological changes that occur during laparoscopy.

The physiological effects during laparoscopy are associated with changes in patient position and the creation of a pneumoperitoneum.

Position (Trendelenburg/Reverse Trendelenburg)

- *Respiratory effects*–in the head-down position the weight of the abdominal viscera causes cephalad shift of the diaphragm with a decrease in functional residual capacity, total lung volume, pulmonary compliance; these pulmonary function changes depend on the patient's age, weight, preoperative lung function, degree of tilt and the intraoperative ventilatory technique.
- *Cardiovascular effects*–the head-down position favours venous return and therefore improves cardiac output; the reverse position causes pooling of blood in legs with reduction in venous return and cardiac output.
- *Central nervous system effects*–the head-down position increases both intracranial and intraocular pressures.
- *Gastrointestinal effects*–the head-down position increases the risk of passive regurgitation.

Creation of pneumoperitoneum

This results in the following:
- Raised intra-abdominal pressure and its consequences.
  - a cephalad shift of the diaphragm, ventilation–perfusion mismatch and carinal displacement with potential for inadvertent right bronchial intubation
  - reduction in cardiac output
  - reduced blood flow to intra-abdominal organs
  - increased risk of gastric regurgitation
- Systemic absorption of insufflated carbon dioxide causing hypercarbia and possible gas embolism.
- Vagal reflexes causing bradycardia and cardiac arrest.

In summary, the extent of cardiovascular changes depends on the intra-abdominal pressure attained, the volume of carbon dioxide absorbed, changes in intravascular volume, patient position, and the ventilatory technique and anaesthetic agents employed.

KEYWORDS: LAPAROSCOPY

5. List, with examples when appropriate, the possible causes of air embolism during surgery and the methods of diagnosis and treatment.

Causes

- Inadvertent intravascular injection of air into vein or artery (iatrogenic).
- Suction of air into open veins or sinuses under low hydrostatic pressures, for example cannulation of central veins especially when the Trendelenburg position is not used; open cerebral sinuses during an operation in the sitting or head up position; open veins and sinuses of the uterus when it is elevated or inverted such as during a caesarean section.
- Entrainment of air with rapid transfusion of blood or infusion of intravenous fluids especially with the use of rotary pumps or pressure bags.
- Reuse of disconnected plastic intravenous fluid bags or use of air vents with intravenous fluid bags.
- The use of extracorporeal circulation such as during cardiac surgery.
- Use of air for the loss of resistance technique in insertion of the epidural needle may be a potential risk for air embolism in small children.

Diagnosis

- Loss or dramatic fall in the end-tidal CO_2 trace of the capnograph.
- Drop in the cardiac output, manifesting as low arterial pressure, weak pulses and poor colour and capillary filling.
- Elevation in central venous pressure with dramatic fall in arterial pressure.
- ECG changes, mainly signs of right-sided strain.
- Mill-wheel murmur heard more clearly when an oesophageal stethoscope is used.
- Precordial Doppler ultrasound.
- Transoesophageal echocardiography.

Treatment

- Prevent further air entrainment by treating the cause, for example:
  - stop intravenous fluid if air is seen in the intravenous fluid system.
  - ask the surgeon to cover open veins or sinuses with saline.
  - reverse sitting or head-up positions. Level (make horizontal) the patient or even make dependent the part of the body where open veins are suspected, for example head-up position when the uterine veins and sinuses are opened or head-down position during insertion of a central venous line.
- Supportive measures, for example increase F_{IO_2}.

KEYWORDS: AIR EMBOLISM

- Aspirate air from the central venous catheter.
- Consider the left lateral head-down position if ventricular flow obstruction is suspected. This may also help aspiration of the air from the central venous catheter.
- In extreme situations, a cannula may be inserted percutaneously into the right ventricle for aspiration of air.

KEYWORDS: AIR EMBOLISM

6. Describe the physiological regulation of cerebral blood flow. Outline how this may be influenced by anaesthesia.

Cerebral blood flow (CBF) should be 50 ml/100 g/min or 15% of cardiac output. It is regulated by:

- *Arterial pressure*
  - Autoregulation: normal brain has the ability to maintain a constant cerebral blood flow despite wide variations in mean arterial pressure (60–130 mmHg). Two or three minutes are required for autoregulation to take place. Mechanisms: myogenic and metabolic; a variety of factors may abolish (ischaemia, trauma, tumours and other intracranial pathology, hypoxia, hypercapnia, volatile agents) or modify autoregulation (hypertension, sympathetic activation). Under normal circumstances regional cerebral blood flow and metabolism are tightly coupled, with an increase in cortical activity leading to a corresponding increase in cerebral blood flow.
  - Cerebral perfusion pressure (CPP) = MAP − ICP ; CPP represents the pressure head available for CBF. Normal is 70–80 mmHg; critical level for cerebral ischaemia is 30–40 mmHg.
- *Venous pressure*–any increase (head-down position, coughing, straining) will decrease CBF.
- *CSF pressure*–raised ICP reduces CBF.
- *Pa_{CO_2}*–hypocapnia reduces CBF and hypercapnia increases CBF; CO_2 reactivity is mediated by hydrogen ion concentration in CSF.
- *Pa_{O_2}*–less influence on CBF than is the case with Pa_{CO_2}; an increase in CBF occurs when Pa_{O_2} falls below 8 kPa.
- *Temperature*–reduction in CBF with hypothermia appears to parallel reduction in metabolic rate.

The influence of anaesthesia is outlined as follows:

- *Drugs*–volatile agents and ketamine increase CBF; thiopentone and propofol cause a dose-related fall in CBF.
- *Disruption of controlling factors*–cardiovascular instability, raised jugular venous pressure (coughing, vomiting, fluid loading, intubation, IPPV), hypoxia, hypercapnia, hypocapnia, hypothermia.

KEYWORDS: CEREBRAL BLOOD FLOW

7. Briefly describe the use of filters in (a) blood transfusion, (b) epidural infusions, and (c) breathing systems.

(a) Blood transfusion

Small mesh filters (20–40 micrometre) have been used in blood-giving sets to reduce the transfusion of microaggregates. Microaggregates may have a role in the development of disseminated intravascular coagulopathy (DIC), but now appear not to be implicated in the development of Acute Respiratory Distress Syndrome. These filters cause a significant increase in resistance to the flow of blood especially after more than one unit has been given. They also cause entrapment of platelets and therefore are unsuitable for transfusion of platelets or fresh blood. Blood filters do not protect against bacteria or viruses. Blood is typically given through a normal intravenous giving set (150 micrometre mesh size).

(b) Epidural infusions

The epidural space has a good blood supply and an efficient immune system. It is, however, in close proximity to the meninges and there is an infection risk. When performing an epidural, one is always at risk of an inadvertent dural puncture. It is mandatory to run an epidural infusion through an appropriate filter. Typically, epidural filters are 0.22 micrometre and are bacterial, and particulate filters.

(c) Breathing systems

Some heat and moisture exchangers (HMEs) are also bacterial, viral, and particulate filters. They are 99.99% efficient but do increase the dead space and resistance to flow. They are widely used for infective cases such as tuberculosis or MRSA and to protect anaesthetic equipment from contamination. Some units only use such filters on high-risk infectious cases but recently there have been reported cases of hepatitis C transmission through anaesthetic circuits and this has made their use mandatory in routine anaesthetic practice.

KEYWORDS: BLOOD TRANSFUSION FILTERS; EPIDURAL INFUSION FILTERS; BREATHING SYSTEM FILTERS

8. Briefly list factors involved in the pathophysiology of septic shock resulting from Gram negative bacterial infections.

Gram negative infections often lead to rapid onset, life-threatening situations. Endotoxins are released and these cause:

- *Factor XII activation*
  - thrombin
  - fibrin
  - clot formation
  - fibrinolysis which ultimately can lead to disseminated intravascular coagulation.

- *Complement and mast cell activation*
  - histamine release and production of kinins
  - reduction in the systemic resistance and leakage of capillaries
  - hypotension
  - reduced renal blood flow leading to oliguria and renal failure.

- Release of myocardial depressant factors leading to high output cardiac failure causing tissue hypoxia and lactic acidosis.
- Endothelial damage resulting in capillary leakage and the acute respiratory distress syndrome.
- Monocyte activation causing fever, and a hypermetabolic state.
- White blood cell activation.
- Free oxygen radical release.
- Arachnoid acid metabolites.

More recently the following substances have been implicated:

- Cytokines
- Tumour necrosis factor
- Interleukines.

KEYWORDS: INTENSIVE CARE UNIT; SEPTIC SHOCK; GRAM NEGATIVE INFECTIONS

9. Outline the preoperative assessment of a patient who requires a partial thyroidectomy. What early complications may result from this operation?

General assessment

The same as for any patient having general anaesthesia.

Specific assessment

To elucidate thyroid status and possible upper airway obstruction:

- *Thyroid function*–assessed clinically and by laboratory investigations. If patient has hyperthyroidism check cardiovascular and neurological aspects; tachycardia, atrial fibrillation and congestive cardiac failure will need controlling in order to prevent thyroid crisis. Other features to look for are exophthalmos, myopathy, diabetes mellitus. Investigations include plasma thyroxine and tri-iodothyronine, TSH, ECG, Hb.
- *Airway*
  - clinical evidence of upper airway obstruction.
  - chest X-ray including thoracic inlet views to assess tracheal compression, deviation and retrosternal extension.
  - indirect laryngoscopy to assess vocal cord function in case of pre-existing damage to laryngeal nerves.
- *Presence of other autoimmune diseases*, for example myasthenia gravis.
- *Presence of superior vena caval obstruction* from a retrosternal goitre.
- *Medication*–what drugs?
  - antithyroid drugs, for example carbimazole; this increases the vascularity of the gland and needs to be stopped two weeks before surgery.
  - iodine–this is sometimes given two weeks before surgery to reduce glandular vascularity.
  - beta-adrenergic receptor antagonists.

Complications

- *Intraoperatively*
  - tracheal intubation may be difficult
  - arrhythmias may occur from stimulation of carotid sinus
  - air embolism
  - pneumothorax.
- *Postoperatively*
  - bleeding
  - airway obstruction from expanding haematoma tracheomalacia, damage to laryngeal nerves

KEYWORDS: THYROIDECTOMY

- hypocalcaemia and tetany
- thyroid crisis.

KEYWORDS: THYROIDECTOMY

10. Write a short account on the normal distribution curve.

In a population or in a large sample of a population the values of many variables, including biological parameters, tend to cluster around a central value, with fewer values spreading on each side of the central value toward the extremes. The frequency histogram or the distribution curve of the values would assume the shape of a bell and is known as the bell-shaped distribution, Gaussian distribution or the normal distribution curve.

Many statistical tests assume that the population under examination is normally distributed. However, because medical studies often use small sample sizes, the assumption that resulting data have a normal distribution should always be tested first. This is especially true when a parametric test such as Student's t test or analysis of variance is applied on a small size sample of data.

The normal distribution curve (see figure below) of the data also has arithmetic benefits. It implies that mean, mode, median and mid-range values are equivalent and that 68% and 95% of the variables lie between one and two standard deviations respectively on both sides of the mean.

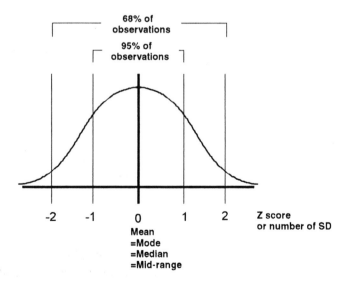

KEYWORDS: NORMAL DISTRIBUTION CURVE; STATISTICS

11. Summarise the problems relating to perioperative management of HIV positive patients.

The problems are summarised under the following categories:

General health

Poor health, poor nutrition, generalised lymphadenopathy, diarrhoea, fevers, malaise, and weight loss are common problems.

Associated diseases

Secondary infections such as respiratory or CNS infections.
Secondary malignancies.

HIV drugs

Drugs used to interfere with viral DNA replication have severe side effects such as anaemia, thrombocytopenia, neutropenia, nausea and vomiting, and peripheral neuropathy.

Psychological problems

Emotional, mental, and psychological disturbances are common. Attention should be paid also to other possible but less common neurological problems such as psychosis, dementia, and encephalitis.

Isolation

HIV patients should be isolated if contamination from their body fluids is likely, for example when there is bleeding or an open wound. Immunosuppressed patients should also be isolated if there is an infection risk to themselves.

Aseptic procedures

Strict asepsis is required to prevent opportunistic infections. The need for using invasive monitoring should be balanced against the risk of sepsis.

Precautions for staff

As it is unethical to test all patients for HIV prior to surgery, it is recommended that universal precautions are applied on every patient as routine.

Simple hygiene: cover wounds and avoid body fluids.

KEYWORDS: HIV; AIDS, PERIOPERATIVE MANAGEMENT

Use gloves, masks and overshoes. Use protective glasses (goggles) and protective clothing if there is a risk of splashing.

Dispose of sharps, avoid use of needles, needle resheathing, or passing needles from one person to another.

Policy for needle-stick injuries must be in place.

Precautions for other patients

Cleaning of theatres is required after treatment of HIV patients. This includes floors, walls and furniture.

Equipment used in contact with body fluids should be sterilised. Disposables should be used when possible, and filters should be used on the breathing circles. Minimum equipment and spaces should be used with induction and recovery in the same operating theatre.

ICU admission

HIV patients requiring critical care are usually managed in an HDU bed with the isolation criteria observed as discussed above. ICU admission may be considered if there is a strong definite indication with a clearly curable condition.

KEYWORDS: HIV; AIDS, PERIOPERATIVE MANAGEMENT

12. Which patient groups are at risk from extravasation injury? How would you manage a case of severe extravasation of thiopentone in the dorsum of a patient's hand.

The patient groups at risk from extravasation injury are:

- The elderly
- The very young
- Patients unable to feel or express pain on injection
- Unconscious patients, for example under anaesthesia or on intensive care
- Those with peripheral neuropathy, for example diabetics
- Patients whose cannulation site is hidden under a bandage
- Patients having multiple cannulation attempts at one site
- Patients being treated by inexperienced personnel
- Patients being cannulated with needles rather than plastic cannulae.

Other factors that may influence outcome are:

- *Site of extravasation.* Sites with little subcutaneous fat such as the dorsum of the hand or with important local structures (for example nerves) such as the antecubital fossa can be particularly devastating. The use of small slow-flowing veins also increases risk.
- *Substance extravasated.* Many drugs are implicated. Some of the worst include most chemotherapeutic agents, most vasoconstrictors, many antibiotics, streptokinase, thiopentone, and etomidate.
- *Volume of substance extravasated.*

General management of extravasation injury of thiopentone into the dorsum of a patient's hand includes:

- *Rapid detection* from pain, and immediate cessation of the injection.
- The provision of *adequate analgesia.*
- *Further management* is mainly based on research performed on chemotherapy extravasation injury but may include:
  - cooling
  - local manipulation of pH.
- *Hyaluronidase.* This enzyme breaks down hyaluronic acid and facilitates spreading of the drug and therefore increase of subcutaneous absorption. This can be combined with saline to aid dispersal and dilution.
- *Wound puncture.* This is sometimes used in premature infants in combination with sterile saline soaks to aid drainage from the subcutaneous tissues.
- *Liposuction.* This has been shown to be very effective in patients with radiographic contrast medium extravasation injury using pre- and post-flushout radiography.

KEYWORDS: EXTRAVASATION; THIOPENTONE EXTRAVASATION

- *Flushout*. This is similar to liposuction but is useful in areas with only small amounts of subcutaneous fat. The skin is punctured at a number of different sites and a large volume of saline is infiltrated below the skin with the use of a special cannula with side holes. The drug and fluid then exit through the puncture wounds.
- *Excision and skin grafting*. In cases of severe tissue injury the only option left may be surgical removal of the damaged tissue.

KEYWORDS: EXTRAVASATION; THIOPENTONE EXTRAVASATION

Paper E

1. Identify the patient groups who are at a high risk of, or conditions that predispose to postoperative deep venous thrombosis. Write short notes on the currently available prophylactic measures.

2. Outline the methods of providing postoperative analgesia for a patient who has had a thoracotomy.

3. List the items that you consider important when submitting a research project to your hospital ethics committee.

4. A general practitioner contacts you requesting information about malignant hyperthermia. Write a letter explaining the condition to her.

5. List the complications that may be encountered when a pulmonary artery flotation catheter is inserted into the left subclavian vein via the infraclavicular route. Choose two complications and describe what precautions you would take to minimise their risk.

6. Write brief notes on the specific problems encountered when anaesthetising for an MRI scan.

7. Outline the anatomy of the oesophagus. List the problems associated with anaesthesia for an oesophagoscopy.

8. Write short notes on the rationale behind the use of preoperative medication for neonates, infants, and children.

9. What are the additives used in red cell storage? What are the complications of blood transfusion?

10. A 30 year-old man is admitted to the casualty department with an acute head injury. List the indications for intubation, ventilation, and referral to a neurosurgical unit.

11. A 40 year-old ASA1 patient is admitted as a day case for an inguinal herniorrhaphy under general anaesthesia. When would you consider him ready for discharge from the day surgery unit?

12. What are the causes of stridor in a child? List the symptoms and signs of upper airway obstruction.

1. Identify the patient groups who are at a high risk of, or conditions that predispose to postoperative deep venous thrombosis. Write short notes on the currently available prophylactic measures.

Patients at risk of, or conditions predisposing to deep venous thrombosis (DVT) are:

- Obesity
- Age over 40 years–risk increases almost linearly with further advancement of age
- Previous history of DVT or pulmonary embolism
- Malignancy
- Major trauma and immobility
- Major operation and lengthy operation
- Abdominal operations, especially in the pelvic region
- Orthopaedic (hip and knee) operations
- Pregnancy and caesarean delivery
- Gynaecological operations
- Combined contraceptive pills and other oestrogen drugs
- Smoking
- Polycythaemia
- Dehydration
- Diabetes mellitus
- Varicose veins.

Prophylactic measures–a combination of more than one measure is usually used:

- Correct any of the reversible conditions above when appropriate, for example stop the contraceptive pill 4 weeks before major surgery and start after 2 weeks if the patient is mobile again. Progesterone-only pill does not require to be discontinued.
- Prophylactic anticoagulation
  - subcutaneous heparin in a dose of 5000 units, two to three times per day is commonly used;
  - fractionated low molecular weight heparin has a longer duration of action and is thought to be more effective in preventing DVT; it is also more convenient to use as a once-daily subcutaneous dosage.
- Mechanical measures
  - elastic compression stockings;
  - leg padding and elevation;
  - manual massage of calf muscles and intermittent pneumatic-pump compression during surgery.
- Regional anaesthesia. The sympathetic denervation, vasodilatation and

KEYWORDS: DEEP VENOUS THROMBOSIS (DVT)

improved peripheral circulation in the legs may reduce the incidence of DVT.

- Early mobilisation after surgery.
- Early screening of high risk patients with the non-invasive duplex Doppler ($>50\%$ of cases are detected in preclinical stage).
- IVC filters.

KEYWORDS: DEEP VENOUS THROMBOSIS (DVT)

2. Outline the methods of providing postoperative analgesia for a patient who has had a thoracotomy.

Postoperative pain is influenced by many factors including age, sex, social class, anxiety, attitudes of staff, and other patients, and includes the nature of the surgery and the type of anaesthesia. It is imperative in surgery such as a thoracotomy to minimise potentially fatal chest complications by providing excellent postoperative analgesia.

The preoperative visit, explanation and discussion of the techniques available is invaluable in terms of future management.

Premedication with opiates and non-steroidal anti-inflammatory drugs may provide some postoperative analgesia.

Systemic drugs similar to those used in the premedication can be given via the oral, intramuscular, intravenous, subcutaneous, or the rectal routes. The mode of administration can be patient- or medical staff-controlled, and the drugs can be given via intermittent or continuous methods. Intravenous morphine PCA pumps or subcutaneous morphine infusions have been used successfully using these techniques.

Regional anaesthetic techniques using "low dose local anaesthetic and opiate" epidural techniques especially in the thoracic region are now successfully employed. Intercostal nerve blocks and wound infiltration have also been used. Intrapleural nerve blocks are also being evaluated as a method of analgesia after this type of surgery.

Miscellaneous techniques with cryotherapy, Entonox, acupuncture, and transcutaneous nerve stimulators have also been tried but have not been found to enhance analgesia in the immediate postoperative period.

The benefits and the side effects of the techniques must be considered. The most common technique in current practice is thoracic epidural analgesia but this has side effects including technical difficulties and drug administration problems, such as hypotension, high block, drowsiness, respiratory depression, and itch. However, this technique provides excellent analgesia which allows for the provision of good postoperative physiotherapy.

Follow-up and constant evaluation of the chosen technique must occur.

KEYWORDS: POSTOPERATIVE ANALGESIA; THORACOTOMY

3. List the items that you consider important when submitting a research project to your hospital ethics committee.

The following is a comprehensive list of the topics that the ethical committee would be interested in when evaluating a research project:

- Title of project
- Names of the investigators and their experience in the field
- Where and when the project will take place
- Objective of the study
- Type of study
  - randomised/controlled
  - case study control
  - single case series
  - qualitative survey
  - retrospective survey
- Scientific background to the study
- Study design
  - measurements
  - sampling sites, for example blood, urine
- Drugs–type, route
- Subjects–patients, controls, volunteers
- Age limits
- Exclusion criteria
- Costs
- Any personal rewards?
- Protection of vulnerable groups, for example those with mental impairment
- Method of recruitment to study
- Consent to study and statement of non-prejudice if refusal occurs
- How to recruit those whose English is not their first language
- Information to general practitioners
- Statistical analysis
- Confidentiality (patient identity replaced by numbers, computer data handling regulations).

KEYWORDS: ETHICAL RESEARCH

4. A general practitioner contacts you requesting information about malignant hyperthermia. Write a letter explaining the condition to her.

Dear Doctor,

Malignant hyperthermia is a rare but potentially fatal complication of general anaesthesia. It results from an abnormal increase in muscle metabolism in response to suxamethonium (a muscle relaxant) or the inhalational anaesthetic agents. It is inherited as an autosomal dominant disorder and there is, therefore, often a history of death or major anaesthetic problems in a family with the disorder.

It is difficult to diagnose during anaesthesia and presents with clinical signs such as masseter spasm, tachycardia, tachypnoea, peripheral cyanosis, and muscle stiffness. It is associated with metabolic signs such as increased carbon dioxide production, acidosis, hyperkalaemia, hypoxia, and hyperthermia. The metabolic changes cause death in the untreated patient. Treatment includes abandoning or terminating anaesthesia as soon as possible, general supportive measures, and specifically the use of the drug dantrolene. All patients who are diagnosed as having this condition will be observed and treated in the Intensive Care Unit.

The condition is more common in males, children and young adults, and those with musculoskeletal disorders. It is helpful to identify patients before anaesthesia is undertaken. This can be done by referring patients with a family history of unexpected problems or sudden death during anaesthesia, and those with increased blood creatine kinase (CK) concentrations. *In vitro* testing of muscle biopsy is the most accurate method of testing for the condition, but this is undertaken only in specialised centres.

Patients who have this condition must inform the anaesthetist prior to anaesthesia, and family members must be investigated. Patients with malignant hyperpyrexia may have anaesthesia but the "trigger agents" must be avoided. If you have any further queries about this condition, or if you have a patient with it or the suspicion of it, please contact me so that I can offer advice and investigate this individual appropriately.

Thank you.

KEYWORDS: LETTER WRITING; MALIGNANT HYPERTHERMIA

5. List the complications that may be encountered when a pulmonary artery flotation catheter is inserted into the left subclavian vein via the infraclavicular route. Choose two complications and describe what precautions you would take to minimise their risk.

(1) Complications associated with cannulating the left subclavian vein are:

- pneumothorax
- subclavian artery puncture with possible haemothorax
- misplaced catheter
- damage to the thoracic duct with possible chylothorax
- air embolus
- infection.

(2) Complications associated with insertion of a pulmonary artery flotation catheter (PAFC) are:

- arrhythmias
- knots in the catheter
- pulmonary artery rupture
- pulmonary infarction.

Precautions for two complications are outlined below.

- *Air embolism* can be avoided. A sufficient degree of head-down, Trendelenburg position should ensure filling of the subclavian vein with blood. All lines and connections should be flushed with normal saline and any ports should have bungs attached. The PAFC balloon should be checked to see that it is intact before the catheter is inserted. The 2 ml of air are unimportant in most adults but may be significant if the patient has an undetected right-to-left cardiac shunt.
- *Arrhythmias* can be minimised by optimising medication and electrolyte balance before the procedure is begun. Throughout PAFC insertion, one person should watch the ECG monitor. Certain points along the catheter's journey may be particularly arrhythmogenic. If these areas are encountered it is usually prudent to withdraw the catheter and try again once the arrhythmia has resolved. It may be possible to pass quickly through the arrhythmogenic area. Either way, it is inadvisable to leave the catheter tip sited at the arrhythmogenic area itself.

KEYWORDS: SUBCLAVIAN VENEPUNCTURE; PULMONARY ARTERY FLOTATION CATHETER

6. Write brief notes on the specific problems encountered when anaesthetising for an MRI scan.

Problems

- MRI scanners tend to be in the basement of the hospital, isolated from other anaesthetic sites.
- Full independent sets of anaesthetic equipment, monitoring and drugs have to be available in the MRI suite.
- The anaesthetic machine has to be separated from the magnetic field.
- The strong magnetic field will affect pacemakers and may dislodge metal cerebral aneurysm clips or metal foreign bodies.
- There are individual problems with monitoring:
  - *ECG*–in general, cannot be used because of interference, artefact and metal components; if definitely required, ECG can be used with electronic filters and the electrodes placed on the peripheries as far out of the scanner as possible
  - *Sao$_2$*–poor signal, artefact, and the presence of metal components again make oximetry difficult in the MRI scanner; if it is definitely required the probe can be placed as far out of the scanner as possible;
  - *NIBP*–safe to use but requires a long hose and the monitor box needs to be away from the magnetic field
  - *invasive BP*–cannot be used because of the effect of the magnetic field on the transducer
  - *capnography*–can be used, but the main monitor box has to be outside the magnetic field; this may necessitate a long piece of tubing, which will provide resistance and time lag.
- Infusion pumps should not be allowed within the magnetic field.
- The MRI scanner is very noisy and claustrophobic. It is very frightening for young children, and they often require general anaesthesia to allow a scan. The noise also creates a problem with hearing monitor signals and alarms.

Solutions

- The patient should be assessed on the ward as normal. The patient should be directly questioned about the presence of pacemakers, previous neurosurgery, and metal foreign bodies or prostheses. A final decision should be made as to whether the scan with general anaesthesia is indicated.
- All equipment should be available and checked before the patient is taken to the scanner.
- The whereabouts of the resuscitation drugs and defibrillator should be known.
- Skilled anaesthetic assistance should be present.

KEYWORDS: MRI SCAN

- The anaesthetic machine and monitors should be placed outside the main scanning room, and the NIBP cuff and the capnography monitor should be connected to the patient.
- Infusion pumps should be placed outside the magnetic field and long manometer tubing used.
- Anaesthesia should be induced outside the magnetic field and the patient then transferred into the MRI on a trolley that can enter the magnetic field.
- A long Bain's system is the breathing system of choice.
- The anaesthetist should keep in constant eye contact with the patient and the monitors.
- At the end of the scan, the patient should be extubated outside the magnetic field and recovered in standard recovery room conditions.

KEYWORDS: MRI SCAN

7. Outline the anatomy of the oesophagus. List the problems associated with anaesthesia for an oesophagoscopy.

Oesophageal anatomy

The oesophagus is a muscular tube with an inner squamous cell mucous membrane and an outer adventitia. It is about 25 cm (10 in) long and extends from below the laryngopharynx to the junction with the stomach which is about 2.5 cm (1 in) below the opening of the right crus of the diaphragm.

The longitudinal muscularis layer is concerned with peristalsis and the "true" muscle layer consists of three constrictors which are arranged in an overlapping fan-like manner.

- Important *features* include:
  - upper sphincter–cricopharyngeus;
  - cardiac sphincter–related to the acute angle of fundus of stomach.

- *Relations*:
  - posteriorly–vertebral column, prevertebral fascia, hemiazygos veins, and descending aorta in thorax
  - anterolaterally–
    - neck–trachea, thyroid, recurrent laryngeal nerves, thoracic duct, vagi, and great vessels
    - thorax–heart, pericardium, pleura, bronchi, thoracic duct, and azygos vein
- *Arterial supply*–branches of inferior thyroid, aorta and left gastric arteries.
- *Venous drainage*–to inferior thyroid, azygos, and left gastric vein.
- *Nerve supply*–oesophageal plexus from sympathetic chain and greater splanchnic nerves, and parasympathetic input from the vagi and recurrent laryngeal nerves.

Specific problems associated with anaesthesia include:

- Vomiting and aspiration
- Patients can be of any age (neonate to elderly)
- Dysrhythmias
- Haemorrhage (in oesophageal varices)
- Unpredictable duration of procedure
- Perforation of the oesophagus
- Shared airway

KEYWORDS: OESOPHAGUS, ANATOMY; OESOPHAGOSCOPY

8. Write short notes on the rationale behind the use of preoperative medication for neonates, infants, and children.

Neonates and infants

Atropine, an anticholinergic drug, is usually required for its antisialogogue effects, as secretions can very easily upset the small airways. Atropine will also reduce the susceptibility to bradycardia because of the high vagal tone in this age group. Sedation is not used in neonates and is not usually required in infants. Presence of a parent is not critical in this age group. EMLA cream is considered only if intravenous induction is planned. The amount used should be kept to a minimum, for example applied to one marked site, to reduce the risk of toxicity.

Children aged 1–4 years (preschool age)

It is often difficult to establish rapport with children at this age because they do not readily co-operate in an unusual environment such as that found in the anaesthetic room. They usually require sedation, for example with temazepam, midazolam or trimeprazine. Atropine acts as an antisialogogue and could be considered for operations where vagal stimulation is anticipated. The presence of one parent is usually very helpful.

Children aged 5 years and over

Preoperative rapport with the child is very important. Intravenous induction or inhalational induction can be explained to the child at this stage. Sedation is optional. The child can be given this choice but it is often not requested! The effect of sedation should be explained to the child as some children may find the experience strange. The presence of a parent is not critical but is usually helpful to reduce any anxiety the child may have.

KEYWORDS: PREMEDICATION FOR CHILDREN; NEONATAL PREMEDICATION

9. What are the additives used in red cell storage? What are the complications of blood transfusion?

Additives

The additives used to promote red cell storage include:

- Citrate–chelates calcium.
- Phosphate–maintains ATP, decreases haemolysis.
- Adenine–maintains ATP, improves cell mobility.
- Saline–decreases viscosity.
- Glucose–energy.
- Mannitol–decreases haemolysis.

Complications

The complications of transfusion are listed below:

- *Physical*
  - overload
  - hypothermia
  - embolism
- *Immunological*
  - pyrogenic
  - type I hypersensitivity
  - graft versus host disease
- *Infective*
  - hepatitis B and C
  - syphilis
  - HIV
  - cytomegalovirus
  - malaria
  - Epstein–Barr virus
- *Haemolytic transfusion reactions*
  - human errors
- *Biochemical*
  - acid/base
  - hyperkalaemia
  - citrate toxicity
- *Disseminated intravascular coagulation.*

The complications of blood transfusion, especially massive transfusion can be serious. The most important factor in the transfusing of blood is to avoid human errors, especially giving wrong blood to the wrong patient.

KEYWORDS: RED CELL STORAGE; BLOOD TRANSFUSION COMPLICATIONS

10. A 30 year-old man is admitted to the casualty department with an acute head injury. List the indications for intubation, ventilation, and referral to a neurosurgical unit

Indications for intubation and ventilation after head injury*

- Immediate:
  - coma–not obeying commands, not speaking, not eye opening
  - loss of protective laryngeal reflexes
  - ventilatory insufficiency as judged by blood gases: hypoxaemia ($Pao_2 < 9$ kPa on air, or < 13 kPa on oxygen); hypercarbia ($Paco_2 > 6$ kPa)
  - spontaneous hyperventilation causing $Paco_2 < 3.5$ kPa
  - respiratory arrhythmia

- Before the start of the journey:
  - significantly deteriorating conscious level, even if not in coma
  - bilateral fractured mandible
  - copious bleeding into the mouth (example from a skull fracture)
  - seizures.

Criteria for neurosurgical referral of head-injured patients

- Without preliminary head CT:
  - coma persisting after resuscitation even without a skull fracture
  - deterioration in the level of consciousness of more than 2 Glasgow Coma Scale points, or progressive neurological deficit
  - open or penetrating injury, depressed or basal skull fracture
  - tense fontanelle in a child
  - if a CT is indicated but cannot be performed within a reasonable time (3–4 hours) in the general hospital
- After CT scan in a general hospital:
  - abnormal CT (preferably after neurosurgical opinion on electronically transferred images)
  - CT normal, but patient's progress unsatisfactory

* From the recommendations for the transfer of patients with acute head injuries to neurosurgical units. Association of Anaesthetists of Great Britain and Ireland, December 1996.

KEYWORDS: HEAD INJURY; NEUROSURGERY UNIT REFERRAL

11. A 40 year-old ASA1 patient is admitted as a day case for an inguinal herniorrhaphy under general anaesthesia. When would you consider him ready for discharge from the day surgery unit?

The prompt and safe discharge of patients from a day surgery unit helps in improving efficiency and reducing costs. The use of discharge criteria and discharge scoring systems ensure safe discharge after anaesthesia. A set of day surgery discharge criteria is described below.

- The patient's vital signs should have been stable for at least one hour.
- The patient must be:
  - orientated to person, place, and time, or returned to preoperative mental status
  - able to maintain oral fluids
  - able to void urine
  - able to dress himself (consistent with preoperative state)
  - able to walk without assistance (consistent with preoperative state)
- The patient must not have:
  - more than minimal nausea or vomiting
  - excessive pain
  - bleeding
- A responsible fit adult should escort the patient home and stay for at least 24 hours.

Discharge scoring systems have been evaluated. A common system in use is the modified Post-Anaesthesia Discharge Scoring System (PADSS). This is based on:

- vital signs
- ambulation and mental status
- pain
- nausea/vomiting
- surgical bleeding

The patient is considered "home ready" when the required numerical score is achieved on two occasions at 30-minute intervals. Any discharge criteria/scoring system must be used with commonsense and clinical judgement, and the patient must feel well enough to go home.

Psychomotor tests and driving simulators can be used to assess a patient's overall recovery. However, these tests are complex, require skilled operators, take considerable time to perform and are generally not useful in a clinical setting.

KEYWORDS: DISCHARGE FROM DAY-SURGERY UNIT; INGUINAL HERNIORRHAPHY; DAY-CARE SURGERY, DISCHARGE

12. What are the causes of stridor in a child? List the symptoms and signs of upper airway obstruction.

Causes

The common causes of upper airway obstruction are:

- Congenital
- Acquired
  - infective
    - epiglottitis
    - laryngotracheobronchitis (croup)
  - traumatic
    - laryngospasm
    - postintubation oedema
    - foreign body inhalation
    - smoke inhalation
  - neoplasms

The most common cause seen by anaesthetists is laryngospasm, but upper airway obstruction from infection is perhaps the most demanding in the emergency situation. The incidence of infective causes has decreased recently because of the introduction of *Haemophilus* vaccination and there has subsequently been a drop in cases of epiglottitis.

Symptoms and signs

The symptoms and signs of upper airway obstruction include:

- Barking cough
- Nature of stridor–inspiratory/expiratory
- Chest recession
- Accessory muscle usage
- Hoarseness
- Nasal flaring
- Drooling
- Sitting upright
- Tachycardia
- Tachypnoea
- Cyanosis
- Drowsiness

In the most acute situation these symptoms can lead to complete upper airway obstruction. Anaesthesia is directed towards treating the cause and bypassing any upper airway obstruction.

KEYWORDS: STRIDOR IN CHILDREN; UPPER AIRWAY OBSTRUCTION

Paper F

1. Outline the management of eclampsia.

2. Outline the management of a brain-dead patient before organ donation.

3. What is PEEP? Outline the indications for and list the complications of its use.

4. Give a brief account on the types of muscular dystrophies and their anaesthetic problems.

5. List the causes of abnormal cardiac rhythms arising during anaesthesia.

6. Describe the systems you know for quantifying obesity. Why are the obese unsuitable for day-care surgery?

7. List the indications for acute haemofiltration. What are the differences between haemofiltration and haemodialysis?

8. List the anaesthetic problems of severe, intractable epistaxis in elderly patients.

9. Draw and label the view of the laryngeal inlet as seen during direct laryngoscopy. Describe the positions that the vocal cords may take up following damage to the laryngeal nerves.

10. Outline with reasons, your technique for anaesthetising a 3 year-old child for removal of a peanut from the right main bronchus.

11. Briefly outline the necessary safety precautions when a patient is anaesthetised for laser surgery to the larynx.

12. What are the problems with monitoring a critically ill patient during an ambulance journey to a neurosurgical unit? How may these problems be overcome?

1. Outline the management of eclampsia.

Eclampsia is a generalised convulsion occurring in pregnancy, labour or within seven days of delivery in the absence of epilepsy or any other disorder predisposing to convulsions.

The initial object of treatment is to control the convulsion. Therefore airway control, oxygen, and left lateral positioning of the pregnant patient, who can be either pre- or postpartum, must be made. A suitable benzodiazepine such as diazepam should be administered intravenously in a dose normally of 5–10 mg as a bolus. Diazepam is not prophylactic in the prevention of further convulsions.

Secondary treatment involves stabilising the patient because this disease is multisystemic in its nature. Therefore blood pressure control and monitoring of the haematological system is mandatory to prevent and treat any clotting abnormalities that may occur. The renal, cardiovascular, and hepatic systems need monitoring as multisystem failure can occur. Should oliguria occur central venous pressure monitoring is advisable.

Attention must be given to the delivery of the fetus and often this is done immediately with general anaesthesia in the emergency situation.

Care is often best undertaken in the ITU or HDU environment.

The prevention of further convulsions is best undertaken by magnesium sulphate therapy. This can be given via an intravenous bolus of 4 g followed by a maintenance infusion of 1 g/h. Neuromuscular, cardiac, and neurological side effects may occur and the level of consciousness, reflexes, and serum magnesium levels must be monitored regularly.

KEYWORDS: OBSTETRICS; ECLAMPSIA MANAGEMENT

2. Outline the management of a brain-dead patient before organ donation.

For all potential donors assiduous supportive treatment is essential to prevent deterioration of organs–this will both increase donation rates and improve graft survival and function. Potential donors should be carefully monitored and corrective measures instituted early. Maintenance of tissue oxygenation, organ function, and metabolic and cardiovascular stability should be pursued as for critically ill patients, until and during organ removal.

The local transplant co-ordinator should be contacted early for advice on donor organ suitability. Blood samples should be obtained for screening for hepatitis antigen and HIV, blood group determination, and tissue typing. For heart and heart–lung donors, a chest X-ray and 12-lead ECG should be obtained.

Haemodynamic support

Hypotension is a frequent complication of brain-stem death. This should be treated with aggressive fluid resuscitation and inotropic support, guided by measurement of haemodynamic variables.

Endocrine disorders

Brain-stem death can precipitate a variety of endocrine disturbances. Antidiuretic hormone, thyroid hormones such as tri-iodothyronine, cortisol, and insulin levels are all reduced. The ensuing diabetes insipidus and hyperglycaemia need appropriate treatment.

Temperature control

Temperature regulation is markedly impaired after brain-stem death because of a reduction in heat production secondary to a fall in metabolic rate, loss of muscular activity, and peripheral vasodilatation. Body temperature should be maintained by insulation and active warming.

KEYWORDS: ORGAN DONATION; BRAIN-STEM DEATH

3. What is PEEP? Outline the indications for and list the complications of its use.

PEEP stands for positive end expiratory pressure and is the application of a positive airway pressure in the expiratory phase of ventilation. It is given in pressures of 2.5–20 cm H_2O. Above this level it is called "super PEEP".

It minimises airway and alveolar collapse and increases compliance by increasing functional residual capacity. The net result, which is the indication for PEEP, is an increase in patient oxygenation and a decrease in lung ventilation/perfusion mismatch. It helps to provide increasing oxygenation of the patient without having to increase the Fio_2 and thereby runs the risk to the patient of oxygen toxicity. Therefore it is used when the Fio_2 is maximal to facilitate adequate oxygenation in a ventilated patient.

It has been suggested that PEEP can prevent air embolism and decrease blood loss but these tenets are unproven.

Complications:

- Decreased cardiac output
- Oliguria
- Raised intracranial pressure
- Increased Vd/Vt (dead space to tidal volume ratio)
- Reversal of pulmonary hypoxic vasoconstriction
- Barotrauma (increased risk of pneumothorax)

KEYWORDS: PEEP

4. Give a brief account on the types of muscular dystrophies and their anaesthetic problems.

Muscular dystrophies are a group of genetically transmitted diseases and are due to an inborn error of metabolism characterised by progressive atrophy of symmetric groups of skeletal muscles without evidence of involvement or degeneration of neural tissue. In all forms of muscular dystrophies there is loss of strength with increasing disability and deformity, but each type differs in the groups of muscles affected and the degree of their weakness, the age of onset, the rate of progression, and the mode of genetic inheritance. Associated medical disorders are respiratory infections, kyphoscoliosis, and cardiac abnormalities.

Types of muscular dystrophies

- *Pseudohypertrophic (or Duchenne) muscular dystrophy* is the commonest type. It starts after the age of two with rapid progression and incapacity in the teenage years, and an early death in the twenties. Cardiac involvement is relatively high.
- *Limb-girdle muscular dystrophy* is less severe than Duchenne dystrophy and occurs later in life.
- *Facioscapulohumeral (Landouzy–Déjérine) muscular dystrophy* is a mild form that occurs later in life with normal life span.
- *Myotonic dystrophy* starts at about the age of 30 years with death before the age of 60. Associated problems are cardiomyopathy, baldness, testicular atrophy, and cataract.
- Other *rare forms* include Becker's muscular dystrophy, distal muscular dystrophy, and ocular myopathy.

Anaesthetic problems

- *Postoperative pulmonary insufficiency and chest infections* are due to muscle wasting, kyphoscoliosis, and maldevelopment of the respiratory muscles. Postoperative observation in HDU/ITU is often indicated.
- *Cardiac arrhythmias* may be due to an associated cardiac lesion such as in Duchenne's dystrophy, or an inappropriate release of potassium such as in myotonic dystrophy. Cardiac arrest has been described during induction of anaesthesia in patients with myotonia. Acute heart failure due to cardiomyopathy is also a recognised complication in patients with myotonic dystrophy.
- *Abnormal reaction to muscular relaxants*: increased sensitivity to the non-depolarising muscle relaxants and difficulty in their reversal are known problems. However, some patients, particularly those with myotonic

KEYWORDS: MUSCULAR DYSTROPHIES; MYOTONIA

muscles, may exhibit resistance to relaxation with anaesthetics or muscle relaxants. Suxamethonium can cause an exaggerated response and excessive release of serum potassium especially in myotonia.

KEYWORDS: MUSCULAR DYSTROPHIES; MYOTONIA

5. List the causes of abnormal cardiac rhythms arising during anaesthesia.

Patient factors

- Pre-existing cardiac disease–ischaemia, re-entrant circuits
- Undiagnosed disease–phaeochromocytoma, carcinoid
- Electrolyte imbalance–potassium, magnesium
- Acid-base imbalance.

Anaesthetic factors

- Hypoxia
- Hypercapnia
- Response to laryngoscopy and intubation
- Pain
- Awareness
- Drugs–wrong dose, interactions
- Hypothermia
- Malignant hyperthermia
- Central line irritation.

Surgical factors

- Reflex responses–eye and dental surgery, visceral manipulation
- Retractors incorrectly sited
- Exogenous adrenaline.

Arrhythmias during surgery are not uncommon and are usually benign. The most common arrhythmias arising during surgery are nodal rhythm and sinus bradycardia.

KEYWORDS: CARDIAC ARRHYTHMIAS

6. Describe the systems you know for quantifying obesity. Why are the obese unsuitable for day-care surgery?

Quantifying obesity

Obesity can be quantified using a number of different systems:
- *Height/weight nomograms.* These allow for differences in sex and build. An ideal body weight for height is calculated and the subject is said to be morbidly obese if their weight is > 20% above the ideal.
- *Body mass index (BMI).* This is the weight in kilograms/(height in metres) squared. Normal is 22–28 and morbidly obese is > 35.
- The *Broca index.* This states that the normal weight (kg) is the height (cm) minus 100 for males and minus 105 for females.
- It has recently been suggested that the *distribution of fat* should also be considered, as abdominal obesity is associated with a much higher incidence of cardiovascular disease than other forms of obesity.

Day-care surgery problems

The obese present a number of different problems to the anaesthetist. Many of these problems make them unsuitable for day-care surgery.

Pharmacological

- The obese have a high percentage of body fat and therefore retain anaesthetic agents that are redistributed to the fat compartment for longer. This may lead to increased length of action of anaesthetic agents.
- Doses that are calculated on a mg/kg basis may result in an overdose of drug. This may cause unwanted side effects or prolong the action of the drug.
- The obese patient with obstructive sleep apnoea may be very sensitive to opioids and sedatives.

Physiological

- *Cardiovascular*–increased blood volume and cardiac output that may lead to left ventricular hypertrophy; hypertension, ischaemic heart disease, arrhythmias, cerebrovascular accidents and deep vein thromboses are all more common in the obese.
- *Respiratory*–decreased FRC; low chest wall compliance usually requires ventilation if patients are to have a general anaesthetic; the obese patient may have obstructive sleep apnoea, Pickwickian Syndrome or cor pulmonale.
- *Alimentary*–the obese patient has a high incidence of hiatus hernia and therefore is prone to impaired gastric emptying and reflux of gastric

KEYWORDS: OBESITY; DAY-CARE SURGERY

contents; a rapid sequence induction with intubation is usually needed if the patient is to have a general anaesthetic; there is often hepatobiliary disease with abnormal liver function and frequently type 2 (non-insulin dependent) diabetes mellitus.

Technical

The obese are:

- often difficult to intubate
- often difficult to monitor
- difficult to cannulate
- difficult to perform local or regional blocks
- difficult to handle–two theatre tables may be required

Postoperative morbidity

The obese have a high rate of DVTs, wound infections/dehiscence, and chest infections. The problem with opioids and with regional techniques often makes the provision of postoperative analgesia difficult. Postoperative mortality is three times higher than in the non-obese.

It can be seen from the above lists that anaesthetising the obese creates a large number of pre-, peri-, and postoperative problems. Obese patients often require a more invasive anaesthetic and need to be observed carefully postoperatively. This makes them unsuitable for day-case surgery.

KEYWORDS: OBESITY; DAY-CARE SURGERY

7. List the indications for acute haemofiltration. What are the differences between haemofiltration and haemodialysis?

Indications for acute haemofiltration

- Renal failure with fluid overload.
- Hyperkalaemia if K is >5.5 mmol/l with signs, symptoms, or ECG changes, or if K is >8 mmol/l.
- Severe acidosis thought to be affecting myocardial performance or in patients with a history of ischaemic heart disease.
- Uraemia producing symptoms.
- Urea or creatinine above an upper limit (for example urea >40 mmol/l or creatinine >600 micromol/litre).

Haemofiltration vs haemodialysis

Haemofiltration involves the passage of solute following solvent through a filter through convection. A crystalloid solution is returned back into the circulation. Haemodialysis involves the passage of solute through a semipermeable membrane through diffusion. Having the dialysate and the blood flowing in opposite directions to each other enhances haemodialysis. The addition of hydrostatic pressure on the blood side of the membrane allows for the removal of water–ultrafiltration.

Haemofiltration is usually continuous and therefore more gently corrects abnormalities. Haemodialysis tends to be performed two or three times a week and creates greater swings in fluid volumes and biochemical values. It may therefore produce hypotension and is not recommended in the septic or critically ill patient. Haemofiltration is usually done through a venovenous or arteriovenous catheter. Haemodialysis is usually done through a surgically created arteriovenous shunt.

KEYWORDS: HAEMOFILTRATION; HAEMODIALYSIS

8. List the anaesthetic problems of severe, intractable epistaxis in elderly patients.

Problems of anaesthetising elderly patients

- Altered volumes of distribution
- Lower minimum alveolar concentration (MAC) values
- Pre-existing disease

Problems relating to the pathophysiology of hypovolaemic shock in the elderly

- *Cardiovascular*–the elderly tolerate hypovolaemia poorly. They are less able to vary peripheral vascular resistance to maintain blood pressure. They need careful, expert intravascular fluid replacement and probably central venous pressure monitoring. They should be fully resuscitated prior to anaesthesia. Hypotension may exacerbate angina. Care needs to be taken with intravascular fluid replacement as the elderly patient can easily be tipped into left ventricular failure.
- *Respiratory*–the patient may have poor pulmonary reserve and decompensate in response to V/Q mismatch due to hypovolaemia.
- *Renal*–the elderly patient may have poor reserve function, and acute tubular necrosis after hypovolaemia can occur.
- *Cerebral*–confusion may be apparent.
- *Haematological*–the elderly may develop a transfusion coagulopathy or disseminated intravascular coagulopathy (DIC), and require fresh frozen plasma, platelets, or cryoprecipitate.

Problems relating to the epistaxis

- It is difficult to assess total blood loss since blood can be swallowed.
- Blood in the upper airway and stomach carries the risk of pulmonary aspiration. An anaesthetic technique involving a rapid sequence induction is used.
- If packing and cauterising the nose has failed, maxillary artery ligation may be needed.
- Postoperative problems, depending on the size of blood loss, the frailty of the patient, and the operation performed, may include high dependency care.

KEYWORDS: EPISTAXIS; ELDERLY PATIENTS

9. Draw and label the view of the laryngeal inlet as seen during direct laryngoscopy. Describe the positions that the vocal cords may take up following damage to the laryngeal nerves.

The figure below shows the laryngeal inlet:

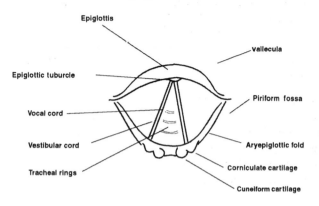

Damage to the laryngeal nerves may lead to the following types of palsies.

Abductor palsy (unilateral or bilateral)

This occurs with partial or incomplete injury of the recurrent laryngeal nerve on the same side or on both sides of the vocal cords. The affected vocal cord (or cords) assume an adducted position instead of the neutral position as the abductors are more sensitive to injury than the adductors. During inspiration the normal cord fully abducts but not the affected cord. During phonation both of the cords, the affected and the unaffected, are able to adduct and meet in the mid-line (see figure below) – the dotted lines represent normal cord positions.

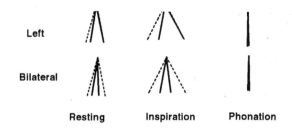

Adductor palsy

Pure adductor palsy is not known to occur.

KEYWORDS: LARYNX ANATOMY; LARYNGOSCOPY; VOCAL CORDS

Abductor and adductor palsy (unilateral or bilateral)

This occurs with a complete incision of the recurrent laryngeal nerve such as may occur during thyroid surgery. Both abductors and adductors are affected. The vocal cord rests in the neutral mid-position. During inspiration the affected cord cannot move to full abduction. During phonation the vocal cords are unable to meet in the mid-line, but in unilateral injury the normal vocal cord may cross the mid-line to meet the affected cord.

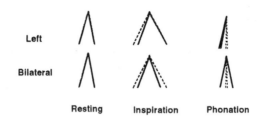

Left   Bilateral

Resting   Inspiration   Phonation

Total paralysis of the cords

This includes paralysis of the cricothyroid muscles (the tensors of the vocal cords) which are supplied by the external motor branches of the superior laryngeal nerves, as well as paralysis of the abductors and adductors supplied by the recurrent laryngeal nerves. The vocal cords assume a mid-position with slack untaut appearance and the anterior-posterior diameter of the glottic opening is reduced. This mimics the cadaveric position of the vocal cords. It is also very similar to the position assumed by the vocal cords during complete muscular relaxation with muscle relaxants.

Resting   Inspiration   Phonation

KEYWORDS: LARYNX ANATOMY; LARYNGOSCOPY; VOCAL CORDS

10. Outline with reasons, your technique for anaesthetising a 3 year-old child for removal of a peanut from the right main bronchus.

This is a serious and potentially fatal situation. ✔

Problems

- The distressed child may be hypoxic, coughing or have some degree of bronchospasm.
- Peanuts are notoriously difficult to remove bronchoscopically as they are smooth sided and fit neatly into the bronchus.
- There is a risk of advancing the foreign body down the airway if positive pressure is applied. This is complicated by the fact that sufficient relaxation of the vocal cords must be produced in order to pass the bronchoscope.
- All the problems associated with general anaesthesia and bronchoscopy are present, for example a shared airway.
- Rigid bronchoscopy is required.

Solutions

Visit the child and parent preoperatively. A full history and explanation must be given to the parents. Assess the degree of urgency. Reduce risks of a full stomach by fasting the child. In the anaesthetic room, having performed all routine checks and preparations, induce anaesthesia using an inhalational induction with oxygen, nitrous oxide, and sevoflurane or halothane. Once anaesthesia has been induced establish intravenous access. The anaesthetic is "deepened" by the use of a volatile agent in oxygen. It is best to use a more soluble volatile agent at this stage and therefore sevoflurane is not recommended for maintenance as it wears off too quickly. Anaesthesia is taken to the deepest level that prudence allows. The mask is then removed and the bronchoscope passed. The patient breathes spontaneously throughout the procedure. Depending on the type of the bronchoscope it may be possible to pass oxygen and volatile agent through a sidearm on the bronchoscope. If this is not possible the child will steadily lighten as air is breathed down the bronchoscope. As the child lightens, the bronchoscope is removed and the process of deepening the anaesthetic is repeated.

KEYWORDS: FOREIGN BODY INHALATION; BRONCHOSCOPY

11. Briefly outline the necessary safety precautions when a patient is anaesthetised for laser surgery to the larynx.

Risks

There are risks to both patient and operating room staff when lasers are used. These include:

- Explosions and fires following ignition of anaesthetic vapours, tracheal tubes, and drapes.
- Ocular damage both corneal and retinal.
- Atmospheric contamination–the fumes produced by vaporisation of tissues with lasers may be noxious, potentially infective, and can cause acute bronchial inflammation.

Safety precautions

- A formal safety programme should be in operation in hospitals undertaking laser surgery.
- Personnel should be properly trained in the use of the equipment and regular servicing carried out to ensure its correct function.
- Notices restricting admission should be posted on the doors to the theatre in which laser is being used.
- Personnel should wear protective goggles to prevent eye damage from deflected laser beam.
- Measures must be taken to reduce risk of fires.
- Shield endotracheal tubes from the laser beam by wrapping with aluminium foil or use a flexible metallic tube.
- Use double cuffed tubes, and fill cuffs with saline which absorbs stray energy more effectively than air.
- Choose an anaesthetic technique that could avoid the use of tracheal intubation, for example injector techniques, high frequency ventilation, cuirass ventilation.
- Use non-explosive mixtures of gases, for example under 30% oxygen in nitrogen or helium.
- Limit laser power and duration of bursts.
- Use saline-soaked swabs to protect surrounding tissues from laser.

KEYWORDS: LASER SURGERY; LARYNX LASER SURGERY

12. What are the problems with monitoring a critically ill patient during an ambulance journey to a neurosurgical unit? How may these problems be overcome?

Problems

- Vehicle movement:
  - affects NIBP, ECG and Sao_2
  - may affect zeroing
  - may dislodge monitoring devices
  - makes clinical assessment difficult and hazardous.
- Moving patient in and out of ambulance may require interruption of monitoring.
- Light may interfere with Sao_2 probe or make screens difficult to view.
- Noise may obscure the noise of monitors or alarms.
- Limited space may make it difficult to see all the monitors together.
- Monitoring less sophisticated.
- Length of journey may be considerably longer than expected.
- Battery life.

Solutions

- Arrange for minimal monitoring requirements to be met–clinical observation and technical monitoring includes NIBP, ECG, oximetry, and capnography.
- Check your equipment and monitors for life of batteries and spare batteries.
- Ensure that you are happy with the "set up" on your unit before leaving. Your equipment should be attached and working and you should have formulated a plan for all stages of the transfer.
- Transfer into the ambulance without disruption to monitoring.
- Once in the ambulance check the patient's condition, do baseline observations and ensure monitoring is functioning properly. Find out where you are sitting and check that you can see all the monitors from that position. It is preferable to insist on a seat where you can easily reach your patient's body and giving sets. Pull all window blinds down to minimise external light. Tape Sao_2 probes to the finger and try to keep NIBP cuffs isolated from any potentially vibrating solid objects, such as cot sides, that may create artefact.
- Negotiate with your ambulance driver the optimum speed for the transfer.
- Be vigilant throughout the journey. Observe the patient's clinical condition and regularly record the observations on a chart. Monitor the

KEYWORDS: TRANSFER TO NEUROSURGERY; NEUROSURGERY UNIT; MONITORING PROBLEMS; AMBULANCE TRANSFER

state of your monitors–do they need a battery change?
- At the receiving hospital the same rules apply. Check that your monitoring is functioning properly before leaving the ambulance.

KEYWORDS: TRANSFER TO NEUROSURGERY; NEUROSURGERY UNIT; MONITORING PROBLEMS; AMBULANCE TRANSFER

Paper G

1. List all the possible factors that may contribute to postoperative nausea and vomiting.

2. Discuss the causes of heat loss during general anaesthesia. What are the physiological effects of hypothermia in the anaesthetised patient?

3. Briefly describe the physical principles involved in capnography.

4. Give a brief account of the structure and nerve supply of the diaphragm.

5. Outline the anaesthetic management of a 36 year-old male undergoing a lumbar discectomy.

6. List the methods of pain relief available to a patient who has multiple rib fractures. Give the benefits and problems of each of them.

7. Outline the management of a "failed intubation" in an emergency caesarean section.

8. Describe the techniques that are available for acute pacing of a patient in complete heart block immediately post-cardiac arrest.

9. Describe the precautions you would take when inserting a chest drain for a non-tension pneumothorax into a 40 year-old female patient known to be hepatitis B carrier e-antigen positive.

10. Summarise the problems associated with anaesthetising patients with transplanted organs.

11. Describe the technique of interpleural block.

12. Give details of the disadvantages and advantages of administering sodium bicarbonate at cardiac arrests.

1. List all the possible factors that may contribute to postoperative nausea and vomiting.

The factors contributing to postoperative nausea and vomiting (PONV) may be classified as relating to the patient, the anaesthetic technique, or the type of surgery.

Patient

- History of previous PONV
- History of motion sickness
- Female–particularly when the surgery is during the ovulation phase of the menstrual cycle
- Pregnant women
- Lower in infants and small children and lower in elderly patients

Anaesthesia

- Fasting. Infusion of intravenous fluids reduces the incidence of PONV.
- Inflation of stomach with air such as during incorrect or difficult mask ventilation.
- Choice of intravenous anaesthetic. Etomidate and ketamine are known to cause PONV. Propofol causes the least PONV. It has been suggested that it has antiemetic effects.
- Choice of inhalational anaesthetic. Ether which is not used today in the developed countries is very emetic. The currently used inhalational anaesthetics are not particularly emetic, but when compared to total intravenous anaesthesia they do have a higher incidence of PONV. The use of N_2O is thought to be associated with an increase in the incidence of PONV.
- The use of opioid analgesics is known to be associated with higher PONV. Simple analgesics and non-steroidal anti-inflammatory drugs have no effect on PONV but their use has a sparing effect on the requirement of opioids and may reduce PONV.
- Inadequate analgesia.
- Premedication with metoclopramide, droperidol, or ondansetron, or inclusion of these drugs in the anaesthetic technique may reduce the incidence of PONV.
- The effect of anticholinergic drugs is controversial.
- Anticholinesterase drugs such as neostigmine are known to increase the incidence of PONV.
- PONV is also associated with deranged physiology such as in hypotension, hypoxia and hypercapnoea.
- Local and regional anaesthesia do not cause PONV themselves, but

KEYWORDS: POSTOPERATIVE NAUSEA AND VOMITING (PONV)

secondary hypotension/hypoxia or inadequate analgesia may be contributing factors.

Surgery

- Laparoscopic procedures.
- ENT operations–PONV is especially high with middle ear surgery.
- Abdominal (intraperitoneal and visceral) operations.
- Ophthalmic surgery, especially with strabismus operation.
- Orchidopexy.
- Ambulatory surgery.

KEYWORDS: POSTOPERATIVE NAUSEA AND VOMITING (PONV)

2. Discuss the causes of heat loss during general anaesthesia. What are the physiological effects of hypothermia in the anaesthetised patient?

Hypothermia is a consequence of anaesthesia and surgery. Heat is lost by radiation, convection, evaporation and conduction. There is also decreased heat production. The physiological mechanisms for conserving heat are also affected by anaesthesia. For example, behavioural techniques and the ability to vasoconstrict are lost and shivering is prevented by muscle relaxants. The main causes of heat loss are radiation and evaporation.

Factors contributing to heat loss

- Cold operating theatre environment
- Prolonged surgery
- Infusion of cold intravenous fluids
- Breathing cool dry anaesthetic gases
- Use of cold antiseptic solutions and cold irrigating solutions
- Exposure of abdominal and thoracic contents
- Patient factors
  - extremes of age
  - associated endocrine disorders
  - severe illness

Effects of hypothermia

- *Cardiovascular*–vasoconstriction, reduced cardiac output, J waves on ECG at 30°C, ventricular arrhythmias at 30°C, ventricular fibrillation at 28°C, increased blood viscosity, increased haematocrit, thrombocytopenia.
- *Respiratory*–decreased O_2 delivery, increased O_2 requirement, apnoea at 24°C.
- *Neurological*–confusion below 35°C, unconsciousness at 30°C, reduction in MAC of volatile agents, cessation of all cerebral electrical activity below 18°C.
- *Metabolic*–reduced basal metabolism, hyperglycaemia, increased fat mobilisation, decreased drug metabolism.
- *Renal*–GFR reduced by 50% at 30°C.

KEYWORDS: HYPOTHERMIA

3. Briefly describe the physical principles involved in capnography.

Capnography is the continuous measurement of carbon dioxide concentration in the expired gases. The widely used method of measurement in clinical capnography is absorption spectrophotometry with infrared light and operates on the principle that the concentration of CO_2 can be determined by passing infrared light of a particular wavelength (approximately 4.3 micrometre) through a very small amount of expired gas. The CO_2 then absorbs the infrared light in proportion to its concentration. The figure below shows the set-up:

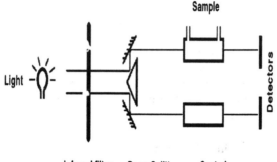

Sample

Light

Detectors

Infrared filter   Beam Splitter   Control

The absorption of infrared light is dependent upon the molecules of the gas being polyatomic and asymmetric, therefore N_2O and water vapour are two examples of gases that can interfere with the measurement of CO_2 as in the figure overleaf:

Corrections for N_2O interference can be programmed into the capnogram by incorporating an additional wavelength of light to measure the concentration of N_2O independently. Single-atom gases such as H_2, H, and Ar, or gases with symmetric molecules like N_2 and O_2 do not absorb infrared light and therefore do not interfere with this measurement.

KEYWORDS: CAPNOGRAPHY

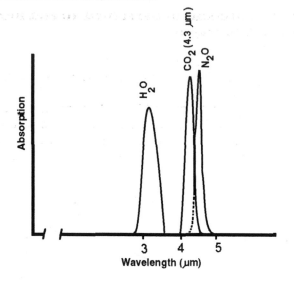

4. Give a brief account of the structure and nerve supply of the diaphragm.

The diaphragm constitutes the great muscular septum between the thorax and the abdomen. It consists of peripheral muscle and a central tendon of strong interlacing bundles which is continuous with the fibrous pericardium above. The right hemidiaphragm is higher than the left. The level of the diaphragm is elevated in late pregnancy, gross ascites or obesity, in the presence of a pneumoperitoneum, and in patients with large abdominal tumours. The drawing below outlines the structures of the diaphragm:

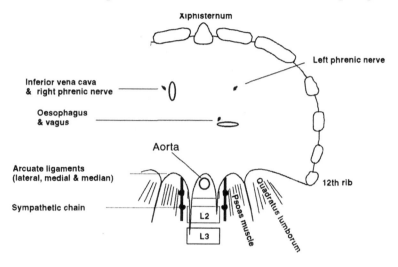

Origins

- Crura (from the lumbar vertebral bodies; the left from the 1st and 2nd, the larger right from the 1st, 2nd, and 3rd).
- Median arcuate ligament (fibrous arch joining the two crura)
- Medial arcuate ligament (a thickening of the fascia over the psoas)
- Lateral arcuate ligament (a condensation of fascia over quadratus lumborum to 12th rib)
- Costa (tips of the last six costal cartilages)
- Xiphisternum (two slips from the posterior aspect of the xiphoid)

Foramina

- Inferior vena cava (at T8 level in tendinous portion of diaphragm)
- Oesophagus, vagi, and oesophageal branches of the left gastric vessels

KEYWORDS: DIAPHRAGM ANATOMY

(at T10)
- Aorta, thoracic duct, and azygos vein (at T12 behind median arcuate ligament)

Nerve supply

- Motor phrenic nerves (C3, C4, C5)
- Sensory–serous surface of central tendon innervated by phrenic nerve (hence shoulder referred pain from diaphragm); peripheral muscular portion innervated by lower six thoracic nerves

KEYWORDS: DIAPHRAGM ANATOMY

5. Outline the anaesthetic management of a 36 year-old male undergoing a lumbar discectomy.

A full history, examination (especially neurological), and appropriate investigations are undertaken. The main problems are intraoperative and these are considered below.

(1) *Prone position.* This leads to several problems:

- Airway: the tracheal tube must not be allowed to dislodge or kink–the consequences are obviously disastrous. Tracheal tubes made of reinforced nylon are available. These do not kink, but often require an introducer for insertion, and cannot be cut down to an appropriate size, thereby running the risk of inadvertent right main bronchus insertion.
- The eyes must be protected because corneal abrasions can occur.
- A "Montreal" mattress, which allows correct abdominal positioning, is often used. Incorrect patient positioning can cause pressure on the abdomen leading to inferior vena caval compression. This can cause a relative decrease in cardiac output. Blood will return to the heart via the epidural veins and this will lead to a haemorrhagic operative site. Pressure on the diaphragm also causes diaphragmatic splinting.
- Specific nerve damage must be avoided. Nerves particularly likely to be affected are the brachial plexus, the ulnar nerves at the elbow, and the nerves of the wrist. Femoral nerve damage has also been reported.

(2) *Secure venous access* is necessary especially when the patient is being transferred to and from the operating table.

(3) *Hypotensive anaesthesia.* Surgeons prefer an avascular field and some wish for hypotensive anaesthesia. Correct positioning of the patient with minimal blood flow through the epidural veins is often adequate irrespective of the blood pressure.

(4) *Infection* is potentially fatal and antibiotic therapy is often routine.

(5) *Postoperative pain relief* is necessary and appropriate discussion must be undertaken preoperatively. Systemic opiates are often necessary.

KEYWORDS: LUMBAR DISCECTOMY; PRONE POSITION; ORTHOPAEDICS

6. List the methods of pain relief available to a patient who has multiple rib fractures. Give the benefits and problems of each of them.

Methods

- Systemic analgesics
  - simple analgesics
  - non-steroidal anti-inflammatory drugs
  - Entonox
  - opioids
- Intercostal nerve blocks
- Thoracic epidural analgesia
- Intrapleural analgesia

Benefits and problems

Systemic analgesia
Benefits
- Non-invasive, simple to administer and does not require skilled operator or anaesthetist.

Problems
- Does not provide effective analgesia. Painful ribs/chest wall due to inadequate analgesia may lead to further respiratory complications such as hypoventilation, atelectasis, and retention of secretions.
- Opioids are probably the most effective amongst systemic analgesics but also carry more side effects, such as respiratory depression, nausea, and vomiting.

Intercostal nerve blocks

Benefits
- Effective analgesia.
- Allows physiotherapy with possible reduction of respiratory complications such as hypoventilation, atelectasis, and retention of secretions.

Problems
- Invasive, requires a skilled and experienced anaesthetist.
- Risk of toxicity of local anaesthetics.
- Risk of pneumothorax.
- Multiple injections.
- Analgesia is short lived and use of catheter is not possible.

KEYWORDS: RIB FRACTURE; PAIN MANAGEMENT

Thoracic epidural analgesia

Benefits
- Very effective analgesia.
- Can be used continuously with a catheter.
- Allows physiotherapy with possible reduction of respiratory complications.

Problems
- Invasive, requires a skilled and experienced anaesthetist.
- Complications as for spinal/epidural analgesia which include dural tap, high block, hypotension.

Intrapleural analgesia

Benefits
- Effective analgesia.
- Can be used continuously with a catheter.

Problems
- Invasive, requires a skilled and experienced anaesthetist.
- High risk of pneumothorax.
- Risk of phrenic nerve and recurrent laryngeal nerve palsies.

KEYWORDS: RIB FRACTURE; PAIN MANAGEMENT

7. Outline the management of a "failed intubation" in an emergency caesarean section.

This is a difficult and potentially fatal situation. Before any general anaesthetic caesarean section is made in the emergency situation, a plan for failed intubation management must be made.

The anaesthetist must know the degree of urgency of the caesarean section. A caesarean section for "severe fetal bradycardia" cannot be delayed whereas "failure to progress" allows the anaesthetist more time to make further decisions. In other words, the decision as to whether a general anaesthetic should be continued or regional anaesthesia be employed should be made prior to commencing the general anaesthetic.

The mother's safety is paramount. The general anaesthetic can be continued with either a face mask or a laryngeal mask and with the patient spontaneously breathing a suitable volatile anaesthetic agent and 100% oxygen. Opiates can supplement the anaesthetic after delivery of the baby. Alternatively the mother can be awakened. After consideration, anaesthesia may be recommenced with senior help and with advanced intubation devices such as a fibreoptic laryngoscope. "*In extremis*" cricothyroid puncture has been successfully used to secure the airway.

If regional anaesthesia is not contraindicated and can be performed, the mother should be woken up, and spinal or epidural anaesthesia commenced. There are potential problems in this situation as high/total spinal blockade will be particularly dangerous because resuscitation is difficult owing to the potentially fatal airway problem.

Specific points of care include:

- Help should be called for early.
- Ideally, cricoid pressure should be maintained
- Hypoxia must be avoided.
- A second dose of suxamethonium should only be given if intubation is deemed absolutely possible and there is no hypoxia.
- Left lateral tilt should be maintained.

KEYWORDS: INTUBATION, FAILED; CAESAREAN SECTION; OBSTETRICS

8. Describe the techniques that are available for acute pacing of a patient in complete heart block immediately post-cardiac arrest.

Repeated precordial chump

This is the least satisfactory option. If other equipment is not immediately to hand, repeated rhythmic striking of the precordium with the fist may produce enough electrical activity in the myocardium to produce depolarisation and contraction. This technique is traumatic and may be ineffective.

External pacemaker

This is available in some hospitals and has the advantage that it can be rapidly applied to the patient and does not require central venous access or radiographic imaging. It involves two pads coated with adhesive electrically conductive gel, connected to a special unit that allows for adjustment of the energy delivered to the pads. In this way, the energy is increased until capture occurs and the patient is successfully paced. Energy is then turned down to threshold as in temporary pacing.

Disadvantages of this technique include:

- discomfort if the patient is conscious
- skin burns from the pads
- usefulness for a short period of time only
- not always effective

Temporary transvenous pacing wire

In this technique a thin, bipolar pacing wire is connected to the myocardium. The wire is initially passed through the subclavian or internal jugular vein and then manipulated into the right ventricular apex with cardiac fluoroscopy. The energy required for pacing is then established by turning the energy down initially until the unit is no longer pacing (the pacing threshold). The unit is usually then set to three times the threshold and put on a demand mode of 60–80 beats per minute.

The disadvantages of this technique are that:

- it requires skill and significant technical support
- it carries all the risks of central venous cannulation such as pneumothorax or inadvertent arterial puncture
- the pacing wire may become detached from the myocardium and fail to capture

KEYWORDS: PACING, TEMPORARY; HEART BLOCK; CARDIAC ARREST

- risk of microshock
- the patient has to be as stable as possible before being taken to the pacing room, which may be an isolated site

The advantages of this technique are that:

- it is generally the most reliable of the acute pacing techniques
- it can be left *in situ* for a long period of time (days) until the patient recovers or a permanent pacemaker can be fitted

KEYWORDS: PACING, TEMPORARY; HEART BLOCK; CARDIAC ARREST

9. Describe the precautions you would take when inserting a chest drain for a non-tension pneumothorax into a 40 year-old female patient known to be hepatitis B carrier e-antigen positive.

This patient has high concentrations of virus in her blood. Anaesthetists and other healthcare workers are therefore at risk of occupational infection through contact with infected blood and blood-stained fluids. This may occur through needlestick and other sharps injury, or through cuts and abrasions in the skin of these individuals.

Precautions must be taken to protect not only staff, but also other patients.

- Anyone undertaking or assisting at an exposure-prone procedure must be immunised against hepatitis B virus and know their immune status.
- The procedure must be undertaken in disposable gowns, gloves, masks, visors and overshoes.
- Equipment in the room must be kept to bare minimum.
- Disposable equipment must be used where possible.
- Needles which have been in contact with the patient should not be resheathed or handed to another person. They should be placed either in a tray or directly into a sharps bin.
- All sharps and other equipment must be carefully disposed of in appropriate bins.
- Contaminated material including clothing should be sealed in bags and labelled as infective.
- All non-disposable contaminated equipment should be autoclaved. Where this is not possible the equipment should be thoroughly washed with detergent and water and left to soak in fresh 2% glutaraldehyde solution or hypochlorite.
- Floors and surfaces contaminated with blood should be washed with a solution of hypochlorite and then detergent and water.

KEYWORDS: CHEST DRAIN; PNEUMOTHORAX; HEPATITIS B; DECONTAMINATION

10. Summarise the problems associated with anaesthetising patients with transplanted organs.

An allograft that is functioning well presents few problems. The anaesthetist must however, be aware of these patients' altered physiology and have some understanding of post-transplant complications.

General peri-anaesthetic considerations

- *Effects of immunosuppression*
  - infectious complications–early nosocomial and late opportunistic infections (CMV, HSV, PCP, *Legionella* commonly)
  - associated neoplasia–especially lymphoma
- *Rejection*. The transplanted organ is most at risk of rejection within the first three months, but rejection can occur at any time. If rejection is suspected, the operation should be cancelled if feasible and the patient referred back to the transplant unit.
- *Adverse effects of immunosuppressant therapy*
  - cyclosporine–renal dysfunction, hypertension, gingival hyperplasia
  - azathioprine–hepatic dysfunction, bone marrow depression
  - corticosteroids–pathological fractures, aseptic necrosis of hip joint, diabetes
- *Altered physiology and pharmacology of transplanted organs*
  - drug metabolism and elimination by renal allografts
  - drug biotransformation and metabolism by hepatic allografts
  - denervated cardiac allografts
- *Transfusion and transplantation*
  - immune sensitisation, blood-borne infectious diseases

Specific peri-anaesthetic considerations

Two examples of specific consideration are listed below.

- *Orthotopic cardiac allograft recipients*–denervated heart. Preload dependence; no response to indirectly acting drugs such as atropine, glycopyrrolate, neostigmine; delayed heart rate responses to hypoxia, hypovolaemia; normal intrinsic Frank–Starling response; accelerated coronary atherosclerosis and silent ischemia.
- *Heart–lung allograft recipients*. Loss of cough reflex–can cough to command, but able to protect airway only when fully awake.

Management

Transplant recipients are very well acquainted with hospital procedures; special care and understanding are required when managing these patients.

KEYWORDS: ORGAN TRANSPLANT

- Avoid unnecessary invasive monitoring.
- Avoid enthusiastic barrier nursing.
- Maintain strict asepsis and antibiotic prophylaxis–flucloxacillin, cefotaxime.
- Maintain immunosuppression.
- Maintain renal function and fluid balance.

KEYWORDS: ORGAN TRANSPLANT

11. Describe the technique of interpleural block.

Indications

(1) Acute pain management
  - open cholecystectomy
  - multiple unilateral fractured ribs
  - post-thoracotomy
  - kidney and breast surgery

(2) Chronic pain management
  - upper abdominal cancer pain
  - chronic pancreatitis
  - post-herpetic neuralgia

Technique

The technique involves injection of a local anaesthetic agent into the pleural cavity either directly at thoracotomy or more commonly via a catheter placed in the pleural space. The block must be performed by trained personnel well versed in anatomical landmarks, safe techniques, and potential complications.

A commercially available kit which is designed exclusively for interpleural analgesia is available. Using a sterile technique, locate a puncture site in the 4th–8th intercostal space in the mid-axillary line. Make a small skin incision with a scalpel blade and introduce a 17G curved tip needle at a 30–40° angle to the skin with the bevel up into the intercostal space just above the upper edge of the lower rib. The stylet is removed from the needle after perforation of the posterior intercostal membrane; which can be identified by the distinct resistance it offers. Attach a well moistened and freely moving 10 ml syringe to the needle, and advance the syringe and needle as one unit. When the pleural space is reached the plunger of the syringe is drawn inward by the negative pressure of the interpleural space. Remove the syringe from the needle and quickly thread the catheter through the needle up to approximately the 5 cm mark. Remove the needle while maintaining the catheter position and fix the catheter in place with an occlusive dressing. Insert the proximal end of the catheter into the catheter/syringe adaptor and attach a 0.2 μm in-line filter; aspirate and inject a local anaesthetic, for example 10–30 ml 0.5% bupivacaine with adrenaline.

Use gravity and positioning to extend the block as required, and perform a chest X-ray after catheter placement.

Complications

- Pneumothorax
- Local anaesthetic toxicity

KEYWORDS: INTERPLEURAL BLOCK

- Phrenic and recurrent laryngeal nerve blocks
- Sympathetic nerve block
- Haemorrhage from lacerated intercostal vessels

KEYWORDS: INTERPLEURAL BLOCK

12. Give details of the disadvantages and advantages of administering sodium bicarbonate at cardiac arrests.

Disadvantages

- Overcompensation may produce a metabolic alkalosis, which may result in myocardial dysfunction.
- The metabolic alkalosis will shift the oxyhaemoglobin dissociation curve (ODC) to the left, reducing oxygen delivery to the tissues.
- Bicarbonate administration may actually worsen intracellular acidosis in the presence of hypoventilation as it dissociates to form carbon dioxide.
- Bicarbonate administration leads to high sodium load.
- Bicarbonate is administered as a hyperosmolar solution.
- Metabolic alkalosis may also reduce respiratory drive by a direct effect on the respiratory centre.
- Hyperkalaemia and hypocalcaemia may occur.
- Bicarbonate is physically incompatible with calcium salts and so its co-administration, in the rare incidences at cardiac arrest when both these drugs are indicated, should be avoided.
- Bicarbonate may inactivate co-administered adrenaline.

Advantages

In certain circumstances, such as the presence of pre-existing ischaemic heart disease, acidosis may adversely affect myocardial contractility. Under such circumstances, with proven metabolic acidosis on blood gas analysis, it may be prudent to start to correct the acidosis and see if there is any improvement in clinical condition. If used in this way, sodium bicarbonate still has a role to play in cardiac arrests.

KEYWORDS: SODIUM BICARBONATE; CARDIAC ARREST

Paper H

1. Briefly describe the technique of stellate ganglion block. What are the signs of a successful block?

2. Outline the methods for producing deliberate hypotensive anaesthesia.

3. Describe the ideal intensive care antibiotic. Discuss how closely vancomycin represents this ideal.

4. Describe the intraoperative anaesthetic management of a 3 year-old child with a penetrating eye injury.

5. Write a short essay on fat embolism.

6. "There is no place for suxamethonium in contemporary anaesthetic practice." What is your opinion of this statement?

7. Write brief notes on the advantages a patient may gain if he stops smoking prior to a major elective operation.

8. List the benefits and problems of the drugs available for sedation of patients on the intensive care unit. What are the indications for muscle relaxation in this setting?

9. Compare and contrast brachial plexus block using the axillary and interscalene routes.

10. Outline the special anaesthetic problems encountered in a patient with a prosthetic heart valve.

11. Describe the management of a massive postpartum haemorrhage.

12. Outline the causes of hypoxaemia in the first 24 hours following surgery. How may its occurrence be minimised?

1. Briefly describe the technique of stellate ganglion block. What are the signs of a successful block?

The stellate ganglion is part of the sympathetic chain and is formed from the fusion of the inferior cervical (C7, C8) and first thoracic sympathetic ganglia. The stellate ganglion provides sympathetic innervation to the face, head, neck, and upper extremity.

Technique

(1) Patient supine
(2) Head extended on neck and looking straight ahead.
(3) Aseptic technique.
(4) Palpate Chassaignac's tubercle (transverse process of C6) at level of cricoid cartilage.
(5) Retract carotid sheath laterally with fingers and raise a skin wheal over the tubercle.
(6) Insert a 4 cm 22 G needle directly posteriorly to contact the tubercle, passing medial to the retracted carotid sheath.
(7) Withdraw the needle 1–2 mm, aspirate, and inject a test dose of 1 ml of local anaesthetic solution (lignocaine 1% or bupivacaine 0.5%).
(8) Presuming no untoward effect from the test dose, inject a further 8–9 ml of solution slowly with regular aspiration.

Bilateral blocks should never be performed.

Successful block signs

The signs of a successful block are ipsilateral

- Drooping of the upper lid (ptosis)
- Pupillary constriction (miosis)
- Reduced sweating (anhydrosis)
- Retraction of the eyeball (enophthalmos)
- Conjunctival engorgement and nasal congestion (Guttmann's sign)
- Increased skin temperature
- Increased lacrimation.

The combination of ptosis, miosis, anhydrosis, and enophthalmos is known as Horner's syndrome.

KEYWORDS: STELLATE GANGLION BLOCK

2. Outline the methods for producing deliberate hypotensive anaesthesia.

Hypotensive anaesthesia is indicated to improve surgical visual field access and to minimise surgical blood loss. It can be provided by both general or regional anaesthesia.

The methods available to assist with these aims include:

(1) *Posture*: gravitational effects from raising the head of the patient assist with better visual access, for example in the ENT patient. Each 1 cm height above the horizontal lowers the blood pressure in that area by 0.7 mm Hg.

(2) *General anaesthetic technique*: a "smooth" anaesthetic without a tachycardia, coughing, straining, or bucking stops any rise in venous and arterial pressures. To this end premedication with a sedative is often helpful and anticholinergics should be avoided as they can cause tachycardia. A technique involving intermittent positive pressure ventilation decreases cardiac output and can lower blood pressure and this may stop straining in a spontaneously breathing patient. Some muscle relaxants, such as tubocurare, have ganglion blocking actions and lower blood pressure themselves. Inhalational volatile anaesthetic agents are useful as many have both cardiac depressant and peripheral vasodilatory effects.

(3) *Specific drugs*: many drugs are available. Labetalol, an α and β blocking agent is commonly used and this can cause postural hypotension. Other direct vasodilating agents such as infusions of nitroglycerine can also be used as supplements to general anaesthesia.

(4) *Regional anaesthesia* is often used to facilitate surgery such as total hip replacement or transurethral resection of the prostate because of redistribution of blood away from the operative site. This is due to sympathetic blockade with resultant vasodilatation.

An intriguing problem is how low the blood pressure should be allowed to fall. It is sufficient to state that it must not fall below the appropriate pressure required for autoregulatory processes to function, especially those of the brain and kidneys. This depends on many factors including age and previous medical health.

KEYWORDS: HYPOTENSIVE ANAESTHESIA

3. Describe the ideal intensive care antibiotic. Discuss how closely vancomycin represents this ideal.

The ideal intensive care antibiotic should be stable in a small volume of solution. It needs to be safe to give as a bolus intravenous dose. After administration, it will achieve effective, safe, and predictable plasma levels. It must penetrate all compartments of the body, including the brain and areas with poor blood supply. It can be eliminated from the body by spontaneously and predictably breaking down into inactive, non-toxic metabolites that are excreted in a predictable and reliable way, even in multiorgan failure. It must be active against all pathogens but be harmless to all natural flora. It would be devoid of all unwanted side effects or drug interactions and should be cheap (or even free).

Vancomycin is a bactericidal glycopeptide and is far from the ideal intensive care antibiotic. It is administered in saline (100 ml centrally or 250 ml peripherally) over 1 hour. Shorter infusion times lead to histamine release and (occasionally severe) hypotension and even cardiac arrest. It has good penetration to most body compartments including the cerebrospinal fluid. It has a low therapeutic index with high plasma levels causing ototoxicity and, more rarely, nephrotoxicity. It is eliminated primarily by the kidneys, with 90% excreted unchanged in the urine. In healthy adults it has a plasma half-life of 6 hours but this may be greatly extended in renal impairment. It therefore requires therapeutic monitoring in order to be used effectively and safely. This all adds to the total expense of what is already a fairly expensive drug. Vancomycin is primarily active against Gram positive organisms. It is active against the methicillin-resistant *Staphylococcus aureus* (MRSA) and with the rising incidence of MRSA infections on intensive care units, its use has become more widespread. A recent worrying development in intensive care units has been the emergence of the vancomycin-resistant enterococcus.

KEYWORDS: ANTIBIOTICS IN ICU; VANCOMYCIN; INTENSIVE CARE UNIT

4. Describe the intraoperative anaesthetic management of a 3 year-old child with a penetrating eye injury.

Anaesthetic considerations

- Need for rapid intubation and airway protection due to potential full stomach.
- Need to protect the eye from a rise in intraocular pressure.
- Need for urgent operation–to assess damage, remove foreign bodies, restore integrity of the globe, reduce the risks of infection and sympathetic ophthalmia.
- Possibility of associated injuries–face, head, chest, abdomen, limbs (especially following explosions).
- Possibility of hypovolaemic shock from associated injuries.
- The paediatric patient.

Intraoperative management

Aim to protect airway and eye.

- Assess the balance of relative risks in consultation with the surgeons. Can surgery be deferred for sufficient time to reduce the risks of aspiration and enable intubation with a non-depolarising relaxant?
- Ensure presence of experienced senior anaesthetist.
- Ensure smooth induction, maintenance and recovery–avoid coughing, straining, struggling, vomiting.
- Avoid drugs that are known to increase intraocular pressure–ketamine, suxamethonium.
- Adopt measures to minimise the rise of intraocular pressure with laryngoscopy and intubation–intravenous lignocaine, alfentanil, or fentanyl.
- Use a technique that has been shown to provide good early intubating conditions without raising intraocular pressure–a described technique is to give fentanyl 2 micrograms/kg followed by vecuronium 0.15 mg/kg; at the first sign of muscle weakness give thiopentone 5 mg/kg and apply cricoid pressure. Intubation can be performed 90 seconds following vecuronium, approximately 60 seconds after loss of consciousness. The stomach should be emptied as much as possible before the end of anaesthesia.

KEYWORDS: EYE INJURY, PENETRATING; CHILDREN, EYE INJURY

5. Write a short essay on fat embolism.

This is a clinical syndrome characterised typically by a petechial skin rash, hypoxia, and mental confusion, one to three days after fractures or operations on long bones.

The pathophysiology involves dispersion of fat globules or droplets from fractured bone, crushed fatty tissues or multiple organ injury (less commonly from other conditions such as pancreatitis, burns, or steroid therapy), into the blood circulation. The trapping of droplets is thought to lead to capillary endothelial breakdown and pericapillary haemorrhagic exudates in the skin, mucus membranes, lungs, and brain. Fat droplets also appear in urine, saliva, or sputum.

The petechial skin rash appears typically over the shoulders, axilla, and upper thorax. Similar haemorrhagic spots may be seen in the conjunctiva and around retinal blood vessels. The pulmonary changes include embolisation, capillary haemorrhagic exudates, and pulmonary oedema causing cough, dyspnoea and haemoptysis. Lung infiltrates may be seen on the chest radiograph; these give it the characteristic "snowstorm" appearance. Hypoxia, cerebral oedema, and cerebral haemorrhagic lesions account for the variable neurologic abnormalities seen in this condition such as restlessness, confusion, convulsions, and coma in severe cases.

Prognosis is usually excellent with supportive treatment. The mainstay of therapy is early diagnosis, fixation of fractured bones, oxygen administration (with IPPV only if there is inadequate ventilation), and careful fluid management to minimise the risk of pulmonary oedema. Evidence for the benefits of steroids in large doses is not conclusive but they have been found to minimise the clinical presentation of fat embolism. The use of heparin and dextrans is controversial.

KEYWORDS: FAT EMBOLISM

6. "There is no place for suxamethonium in contemporary anaesthetic practice." What is your opinion of this statement?

This is a controversial statement and arises from the fact that there are many problems with the drug. There are, however, advantages which still make it a much used drug.

Advantages

- Fastest onset of relaxation
- Shortest duration relaxant.

Disadvantages

- Myalgia
- Bradycardia
- Raised intracranial pressure
- Raised intraocular pressure
- Raised intragastric pressure
- Allergic reactions–anaphylaxis
- Hyperkalaemia in burns, paraplegias, and some myopathies
- Prolonged duration in pseudocholinesterase deficiency
- Malignant hyperpyrexia

The side effects range from mild to potentially fatal in nature. Conventional practitioners are of the opinion that the speed of onset and offset makes suxamethonium the most useful agent for those at risk of regurgitation. Many of the common side effects can be prevented by pretreatment with drugs but it must be emphasised that the rare side effects are potentially life threatening.

KEYWORDS: SUXAMETHONIUM; EMERGENCY ANAESTHESIA

7. Write brief notes on the advantages a patient may gain if he stops smoking prior to a major elective operation.

Stopping smoking has been shown to benefit patients before elective surgery.

Hours

If smoking is stopped for longer than 12 hours the carboxyhaemoglobin levels fall significantly. This increases oxygen delivery to the tissues and makes pulse oximetry more accurate. The levels of carboxyhaemoglobin in heavy smokers may reduce oxygen carrying capacity by 25%.

A similar period of abstinence from smoking produces a significant reduction in nicotine levels. The effect of this is to reduce heart rate and peripheral vascular resistance. Nicotine also increases coronary vascular resistance and even short periods of abstinence may improve symptoms of angina.

Months

If smoking is stopped for two months, the mucociliary elevator in the airway will recover and there will be improved clearance of secretions from the tracheobronchial tree.

Depression of immune function that is seen with smoking will also recover over a similar time period.

Variable time course

Some improvement in obstructive airways disease may be seen after several weeks of stopping smoking.

Irreversible

Some of the damage from smoking such as atherosclerosis or chronic obstructive airways disease may be irreversible.

Conclusion

It can be seen that stopping smoking for 12 hours would be important in any patient group in which peripheral or myocardial oxygen delivery is critical. It should be encouraged for all elective procedures. Abstinence for this short period of time has little impact on postoperative respiratory morbidity and mortality.

In patients at risk from postoperative respiratory complications (for

KEYWORDS: SMOKING

example pre-existing respiratory disease, upper abdominal or thoracic procedures), it would be strongly advisable to stop them smoking two months prior to surgery. There is a six-fold increase in postoperative respiratory morbidity in smokers compared to non-smokers.

KEYWORDS: SMOKING

8. List the benefits and problems of the drugs available for sedation of patients on the intensive care unit. What are the indications for muscle relaxation in this setting?

Sedatives

The five commonly used sedative drugs are analysed below.

Propofol

- Benefits–short half-life, no accumulation.
- Problems–hypotension, hyperlipidaemia (paediatrics), product licence, cost.

Midazolam

- Benefits–rapid onset of action, short half-life of the drug and its α-hydroxy metabolite, reversal agent available (flumazenil), cheap.
- Problems–cardiovascular depression, action may be prolonged in the critically ill.

Morphine

- Benefits–cheap, antitussive, reversal agent (naloxone) available, analgesia.
- Problems–slow onset of action, accumulation of morphine and morphine-6-glucuronide (a highly active metabolite) if renal function is impaired, antitussive, delayed gastric emptying and reduced intestinal motility, tolerance.

Alfentanil

- Benefits–reversal agent (naloxone) available.
- Problems–accumulation may occur if hepatic function is impaired.

Ketamine

- Benefits–raises arterial blood pressure, bronchodilator, analgesia.
- Problems–raises intracranial and intraocular pressure, may produce hallucinations.

Indications for the use of muscle relaxants

The routine use of muscle relaxants is not advocated because of awareness and the obvious dangers of airway disconnection. The indications include:

- to facilitate intubation
- to aid ventilation in, for example fighting the ventilator which causes

KEYWORDS: MUSCLE RELAXANTS; INTENSIVE CARE UNIT; SEDATION

complications such as pneumothorax
- to allow the use of certain modes of ventilation, for example pressure controlled ventilation
- in severe hypoxia or hypercapnoea
- raised ICP
- tetanus

KEYWORDS: MUSCLE RELAXANTS; INTENSIVE CARE UNIT; SEDATION

9. Compare and contrast brachial plexus block using the axillary and interscalene routes.

Complications of brachial plexus block

- Phrenic nerve block is common with the interscalene approach. This approach is therefore not recommended for bilateral blocks or in patients with poor respiratory reserve.
- Horner's syndrome is also common in the interscalene group, and rare in the axillary group.
- Recurrent laryngeal nerve block is possible with the interscalene approach and may produce hoarseness. Recurrent laryngeal nerve block is another good reason to avoid bilateral interscalene approaches.
- Intravenous injection is more common using the axillary approach.
- Intra-arterial injection is more common using the axillary approach. It is often found that this technique leads to puncture of the axillary artery with subsequent haematoma formation. If puncture is suspected, this can be minimised with pressure to the puncture site.
- Pneumothorax is rare with interscalene blocks and virtually unheard of with axillary blocks. Pneumothorax is a more common complication of the third type of brachial plexus block, the supraclavicular block.
- Vertebral artery injection is a rare, reported complication of interscalene block and may result in convulsions.
- Intraspinal injection is a rare, reported complication of interscalene block.
- Intraneural injection or other nerve injury is thought to be more common in axillary blocks. This tends to be more to do with the technique employed, or limb malposition, or failure to recognise compression from an expanding haematoma, than with the anatomical site used. Performing the block with the patient awake or the use of a nerve stimulator reduces the risk of inadvertent intraneural injection.

Clinical uses of brachial plexus block

- *Interscalene block*–good for proximal procedures on the arm. Cervical plexus block is also achieved making this technique suitable for shoulder procedures. This technique often fails to block C8 and T1 roots and therefore makes it less suitable for hand surgery, and it does not block the intercostobrachial nerve which supplies the superomedial surface of the upper arm.
- *Axillary block*–this is a useful technique for hand surgery. The musculocutaneous nerve may not be blocked, resulting in an unblocked segment on the radial side of the forearm. The musculocutaneous nerve is usually

KEYWORDS: BRACHIAL PLEXUS BLOCK

blocked if a large volume of local anaesthetic is injected and then massaged in a proximal direction, up the sheath. This technique also fails to block the intercostobrachial nerve, which needs to be blocked separately.

KEYWORDS: BRACHIAL PLEXUS BLOCK

10. Outline the special anaesthetic problems encountered in a patient with a prosthetic heart valve.

There are two fundamental questions with respect to artificial heart valves:
- Is the valve functioning well?
- What is the nature of the valve–mechanical or tissue?

Mechanical valves

- Valve failure is rare; if failure occurs, it is generally sudden and frequently results in the death of the patient.
- Incidence of thromboembolism is high and patients require long-term anticoagulation with the INR maintained between 3–4.5. The risk is greatest with mitral valves.

Tissue valves

- Failure is common, but gradual in onset. A recurrence of cardiac symptoms and signs would suggest that the valve is not functioning adequately, and echocardiography is indicated prior to anaesthesia.
- Thromboembolic complication rate is low and there is no requirement for long-term anticoagulation.

Anticoagulation

The management of anticoagulation prior to surgery demands careful consideration of the clinical risk of bleeding versus the risk of thrombosis. For elective surgery:

- stop warfarin 3 days preoperatively and start heparin infusion 24 hours later (approx 15 000 units/12 hours), maintaining APTT at 2–3 times normal.
- stop heparin 6 hours preoperatively and check INR and APTT 1 hour preoperatively.
- restart heparin infusion 6–12 hours postoperatively and continue until the patient is able to take warfarin.

In the emergency situation fresh frozen plasma may be necessary. For optimal management of such patients advice from haematologists is often required.

Antibiotic prophylaxis

This is essential because prosthetic valves are very prone to endocarditis, which frequently results in the development of a paraprosthetic leak, with consequent haemodynamic deterioration. Intravenous amoxycillin 1 g

KEYWORDS: PROSTHETIC HEART VALVE; ANTICOAGULATION

must be given at induction and continued postoperatively; if the patient is penicillin-allergic, then intravenous vancomycin 1 g or teicoplanin 400 mg should be substituted for amoxycillin.

Intravenous gentamicin 120 mg must be added when sepsis and contamination are likely complications of surgery (dental, genitourinary, obstetric, gynaecological, and gastrointestinal surgery).

KEYWORDS: PROSTHETIC HEART VALVE; ANTICOAGULATION

11. Describe the management of a massive postpartum haemorrhage.

(1) Does the patient have a pulse? If not start external cardiac massage.

(2) Ensure adequate venous access. A 14 or 16 G cannula should be sited in each arm.

(3) Give 60% oxygen via a fixed performance mask.

(4) Connect monitoring NIBP, Sao_2, and ECG.

(5) Call for help: obstetricians, senior anaesthetist.

(6) Alert haematology laboratory and send off blood for FBC, clotting screen, fibrin degradation products/d-dimers and cross-match 10 units.

(7) Record blood loss.

(8) Give 10 units syntocinon intravenously.

(9) Start syntocinon infusion at 10 U/h. Consider intrauterine prostaglandin $F_2\alpha$.

(10) Review the situation with the obstetrician.
- Is there genital tract trauma?
- Is there uterine inversion?
- Is the uterus empty?
- Does the patient require a manual removal of placenta or evacuation of retained products of conception?

(11) If removal of the placenta is required, give 30 ml of oral 0.3 M sodium citrate. Make decisions regarding the suitability of general or regional anaesthesia.
- Epidural and spinal anaesthesia may cause vasodilatation and hypotension superimposed upon hypovolaemia.
- General anaesthesia must be considered with the use of a "rapid sequence induction" technique to reduce the risk of pulmonary aspiration.

(12) Fluid replacement—initially give colloid. Treating haemodynamic values may be misleading as even moderately severe haemorrhage is sometimes manifested only as a tachycardia. Try to keep up with blood volume lost. If, after 2000 ml of colloid, further fluid is required urgently and the laboratory has not yet cross-matched the patient, consider giving type-specific blood or O negative packed red blood cells. Once blood is available, continue replacing losses with blood. Be aware of all the problems associated with massive blood transfusion such as hypothermia and coagulopathy. Repeat the blood tests regularly and correct any abnormalities with blood products.

(13) Once the operation has finished, it may be appropriate to transfer the patient to the intensive care unit.

KEYWORDS: POSTPARTUM HAEMORRHAGE; OBSTETRICS

12. Outline the causes of hypoxaemia in the first 24 hours following surgery. How may its occurrence be minimised?

Causes of hypoxaemia

- *Low inspired oxygen concentration*
  - depleted oxygen supply; delivery system disconnection.
- *Hypoventilation*
  - airway obstruction; central depression from anaesthetic drugs and opioids; residual neuromuscular blockade; sleep apnoea; lack of respiratory drive; pain; diaphragmatic splinting; pneumothorax.
- *Diffusion hypoxia*
  - usually observed as the patient is emerging from an anaesthetic where nitrous oxide is a component; rapid outpouring of insoluble nitrous oxide can displace alveolar oxygen, resulting in hypoxia.
- *Ventilation/perfusion mis-match and shunt*
  - atelectasis; bronchial intubation; pneumonia; bronchospasm; mucus plugging; pulmonary oedema; pulmonary aspiration; pulmonary embolism.
- *Reduction in cardiac output/oxygen carrying capacity.*
- *Increased oxygen consumption–shivering*
- *Diffusion impairment*
  - pulmonary fibrosis, pulmonary oedema; ARDS.

Prevention

Direct prevention at the cause.

- Give chest physiotherapy for at risk groups, for example elderly, obese, bronchitic patients, smokers.
- Administer 100% oxygen on cessation of anaesthesia.
- Optimise oxygen delivery–treat anaemia; improve cardiac output.
- Provide adequate pain control.
- Optimise ventilation–perfusion relationships (CPAP, PEEP, IPPV).
- Decrease oxygen consumption from shivering.

KEYWORDS: HYPOXAEMIA

Paper I

1. Write a short account on the intracellular pathophysiology of malignant hyperpyrexia. How does dantrolene work?

2. A 40-year-old ASA1 patient is ready for discharge from the day-surgery unit after an inguinal herniorrhaphy under general anaesthesia. What would you ensure he receives prior to discharge?

3. Write a short account on the nerve supply of the larynx. Give examples from anaesthetic practice on how this nerve supply may be interrupted accidentally or intentionally.

4. Outline the management of ventricular tachycardia arising during induction of anaesthesia.

5. Describe your management of a 38 year-old HIV-positive male suffering from atypical pneumonia and respiratory failure.

6. What are the problems associated with providing anaesthesia for a known intravenous drug abuser?

7. Outline the causes, signs, and symptoms of acute water intoxication following surgery. What tests confirm the diagnosis?

8. Write a short essay on paracetamol intoxication.

9. Describe how brain-stem death is confirmed.

10. Compare and contrast the use of systemic opioids and thoracic epidural bupivacaine administration for postoperative analgesia following elective surgery for abdominal aortic aneurysm surgery.

11. Outline the intraoperative problems that may occur during elective surgery for an infrarenal abdominal aortic aneurysm.

12. List the nerves blocked during an ankle block and indicate where they may be blocked. What are the complications associated with this block?

1. Write a short account on the intracellular pathophysiology of malignant hyperpyrexia. How does dantrolene work?

Malignant hyperpyrexia (MH) is an autosomal dominant subclinical myopathy in which the muscle fibres show no defect in histology but undergo abnormal contracture responses after exposure to triggers such as volatile anaesthetics or suxamethonium. The main feature of the pathophysiology is an inability to control calcium ion concentrations within the intracellular compartment of the muscle fibre.

Normally depolarisation travels from the end-plate through the transverse tubule (TT) and to the sarcoplasmic reticulum (SR). The SR releases calcium ions which remove the troponin complex inhibition of the contractile elements and cause contraction. Reuptake of calcium is rapidly carried out by intracellular calcium pumps which transfer calcium back into the SR, facilitating relaxation.

In MH there seems to be an excitation–contraction coupling defect which initiates an early surge in free myoplasmic calcium leading to a low threshold and subsequent increased release of ionised calcium at the SR, the so called "calcium-induced calcium release". In the acute attack, the rapid rise of calcium forces the muscle into a disorganised non-propagated prolonged contracture rather than the normal, reversible propagated contraction. The rapid rise of aerobic and anaerobic metabolism, glycolysis, neutralisation of hydrogen ions, and hydrolysis of high-energy phosphate compounds, cause intense heat and carbon dioxide production, lactate accumulation, metabolic acidosis, and release of potassium, creatinine kinase and myoglobulin. A cascading cycle of increasing metabolism, heat, and acidosis results in metabolic exhaustion and breakdown of cellular permeability, leading to muscular and generalised oedema.

The exact aetiology of MH is unknown, but close associations with this condition are specific genetic alterations in two important intracellular receptors: the dihydropyridine receptors which are located in the TT and control the transfer of depolarisation from the TT to the SR, and, more importantly, the ryanodine receptors which are located in the SR and are known to control the calcium releasing channels.

Dantrolene

Dantrolene stabilises the cell membrane and the intracellular excitation–contraction coupling. It binds to the TT and the sarcoplasmic reticulum and reduces the rate and amount of release of calcium ions but it does not affect its reuptake. Dantrolene does not interfere with the transmission at the neuromuscular junction.

KEYWORDS: MALIGNANT HYPERPYREXIA; DANTROLENE

143

2. A 40 year-old ASA1 patient is ready for discharge from the day-surgery unit after an inguinal herniorrhaphy under general anaesthesia. What would you ensure he receives prior to discharge?

A patient who has received anaesthetic drugs must be given the following items.

- *Written instructions*–information sheets should be succinct and easily understood. They should include:
  - General safety instructions to be observed for at least 24 hours. They should not: drive a car or motorbike or ride a bicycle; drink any wine, beer or spirits; make important decisions or sign important papers; travel alone by public transport; cook or use hazardous machinery; engage in sport, heavy work, or heavy lifting; take sedative drugs that are not authorised by a medical practitioner.
  - Specific instructions relating to their surgery. This should include: postoperative care of wound site, activity, follow-up arrangements, anticipated return to work.

- A supply of *take-home analgesia*–full verbal and written instructions should be given about the appropriate administration of the analgesic drugs supplied including possible side effects.

- A *contact telephone number*, both day-time and after-hours.

- A *letter to his general practitioner*–this should state the operation performed, anaesthesia type, discharge drugs, instructions, and any complications that may have occurred; if, however, there is a computer network available to the surgery, this information can be transferred from the day-surgery unit at patient discharge.

KEYWORDS: DISCHARGE FROM DAY-SURGERY UNIT; INGUINAL HERNIORRHAPHY; DAY-CARE SURGERY

3. Write a short account on the nerve supply of the larynx. Give examples from anaesthetic practice on how this nerve supply may be interrupted accidentally or intentionally.

The vagus nerve provides the larynx with all of its nerve supply through two branches on each side, the superior laryngeal nerve and the recurrent laryngeal nerve.

The superior laryngeal nerve travels deep to the internal and external carotid arteries and divides into two branches: (a) the external motor branch which provides the motor supply to the cricothyroid muscles, the tensors of the vocal cords, and (b) the internal sensory branch which carries the sensory fibres from the upper part of the larynx including the vocal cords.

The recurrent laryngeal nerve originates as the vagus nerve crosses the subclavian artery on the right side and the aortic arch on the left side. It runs in the groove between the oesophagus and the trachea on each side of the neck to reach the larynx. It carries both motor and sensory fibres providing motor supply to all of the larynx (excluding the cricothyroid muscles) and sensation from the lower part of the larynx below the vocal cords.

The recurrent laryngeal nerve may be blocked unintentionally by the local anaesthetic instilled during stellate ganglion block, or interscalenus or supraclavicular brachial plexus block. This nerve may also be accidentally cut or injured during thyroid surgery. The superior laryngeal nerve may be blocked on both sides by local anaesthetic to facilitate intubation during awake fibroscopy. This is achieved by blocking the sensory input from the upper part of the larynx including the vocal cords which travels through the internal branch fibres of the superior laryngeal nerve as explained above.

KEYWORDS: LARYNX ANATOMY; NERVE SUPPLY TO LARYNX

4. Outline the management of ventricular tachycardia arising during induction of anaesthesia.

Is there cardiac output?

Check the central pulses. If absent treat as cardiac arrest with cardiopulmonary resuscitation, cycles of DC defibrillation, and administration of adrenaline. If central pulses are present, assess circulation and cardiac output by checking colour, capillary filling, peripheral pulses, and measurement of arterial pressure.

What is the cause?

Check and reverse any secondary causes for ventricular tachycardia (VT). Check the patency of airway, position of tracheal tube, and the adequacy of oxygenation and ventilation. Observe the colour of the skin, the Sao_2 reading (if there is adequate pulse signal!) and the $Etco_2$ if a capnogram is connected. Aim for maintaining a patent airway, adequate ventilation, oxygenation with Sao_2 >94%, and normocapnia.

Treat the VT

In unstable VT (low cardiac output judged by hypotension, weak pulses, and poor colour and capillary filling), urgent treatment should be considered with synchronised DC shock. A low voltage synchronised DC cardioversion should be used and repeated with stepped increase in energy starting with 25 J, and gradually increasing to 50, 100, 150 and 200 J until the cardioversion is achieved. In severe resistant cases consider overdrive cardiac pacing.

In stable VT, one or more of the following medical regimes may be considered; lignocaine 100 mg (or 1 mg/kg) intravenously, repeated in 10–15 minutes and followed by intravenous infusion 1–2 mg/kg/h; procainamide 100 mg (or 1 mg/kg) intravenously, repeated every minute to a maximum of five doses; or amiodarone 500 mg (or 2 mg/kg in children) intravenously given over 30 minutes through a central venous line.

KEYWORDS: VENTRICULAR TACHYCARDIA

5. Describe your management of a 38-year-old HIV-positive male suffering from atypical pneumonia and respiratory failure.

- Does the patient require ventilation?
- Does the patient fulfil local criteria for intensive care admission?
- What is the causative agent?

The first two questions need to be dealt with rapidly and are usually easy to answer. If the patient is looking exhausted or has worsening blood gases, and other forms of respiratory support, including pharmacotherapy, have failed, then he will require ventilation. As the patient is defined as being HIV-positive and not as having AIDS, this is the first AIDS-defining illness. Under these circumstances, he would generally fulfil the local criteria for admission to most units. Once an AIDS patient presents with a further atypical pneumonia, having already been fully treated for a previous pneumonia, admission criteria become more complicated.

Contact with the patient should be performed observing "universal precautions". This involves the wearing of gloves for all contact with body fluids, goggles and masks if fluids may become airborne, and gowns if there is a risk of being splashed.

If ventilation is indicated the patient is induced in a standard way, for example pre-oxygenation, propofol, and suxamethonium, and the airway secured. Initially, simple ventilator settings such as SIMV may be adequate. This may have to be adjusted, for example using high F_{IO_2} levels, PEEP, inverse I:E ratios, or more sophisticated ventilator modes, in order to ventilate the patient satisfactorily. The aim is to support the patient through the acute phase of the illness, while the antimicrobial agents start to work. There are usually special protocols for management of blood samples, including blood gases. These are usually kept to the minimum and sent to the laboratory, rather than analysed on benchtop equipment in the intensive care unit. Continual oximetry is very useful in these circumstances.

A wide range of pathogens cause atypical pneumonia in patients infected with the HIV virus: 50% are caused by *Pneumocystis carinii*, and 50% are caused by fungi, viruses (such as cytomegalovirus), mycobacter, and pyrogenic bacteria such as streptococci and staphylococci. Making the correct diagnosis can have an important bearing on the success of treatment. Pneumocystis is characterised by dyspnoea, little in the way of clinical signs and a chest X-ray that may be anything from normal to showing diffuse alveolar infiltrates. The patient's general condition may look much worse than the chest X-ray. This diagnosis is confirmed by positive identification in sputum, or bronchoalveolar lavage, or brushings. It is

KEYWORDS: HIV; AIDS; NOSOCOMIAL PNEUMONIA; RESPIRATORY FAILURE preferable to take brushings or samples for culture before starting empirical, antimicrobial therapy. If the patient's condition allows, it is also better to wait for results and treat specific, identified pathogens. Often this is not possible and an empirical approach to treatment is required. It is typically treated with high doses of methylprednisolone and high doses of co-trimoxazole.

KEYWORDS: HIV; AIDS; NOSOCOMIAL PNEUMONIA; RESPIRATORY FAILURE

6. What are the problems associated with providing anaesthesia for a known intravenous drug abuser?

There are a number of problems associated with anaesthetising a known intravenous drug abuser.

- *Altered pharmacology*. The patient may have significant tolerance to opiates, barbiturates, or benzodiazepines.
- *Poor nutritional state*. The patient may have a very low serum albumin level and this will affect the amount of free drug available for certain drugs. The patient may also have a very low body fat percentage and this will mean that drugs may be distributed in an unpredictable fashion.
- *Difficult venous access*.
- *High risk case* for hepatitis B, hepatitis C and HIV.
- *Protecting the patient*. The patient may be debilitated or immunosuppressed and is therefore at risk of developing a nosocomial illness. Strict adherence to normal hygienic practice must be observed in order to avoid this.
- *Universal precautions to protect oneself*. Gloves should be worn whenever there is a risk of contact with body fluids; a mask and goggles when there is a risk of fluids becoming airborne, and a gown when there is a risk of being splashed with body fluids.
- *Protecting other patients*. It is important that as much of the equipment to be used should be for single use and be disposable. Ventilators should be protected with disposable bacterial and viral filters. The anaesthetic should be induced in theatre and at the end of the procedure the theatre cleaned according to local policy. Staff in theatre should be kept to a minimum.
- *Protecting other staff members*. Contaminated sharps should be dealt with in a safe way. Body fluid spills should be cleaned up immediately in a safe way.
- *Other infections*, for example respiratory infections, endocarditis.
- The *concomitant use of other substances* of abuse including cigarettes, alcohol, other schedule A or schedule B drugs, and all the physical and mental problems associated with their use.

KEYWORDS: INTRAVENOUS DRUG ABUSE

7. Outline the causes, signs, and symptoms of acute water intoxication following surgery. What tests confirm the diagnosis?

Acute water intoxication occurs after surgery in which irrigating fluid (commonly glycine) has been used in association with a diathermy. Water is absorbed into any open venous sinuses and the symptoms can appear within 15 minutes from the start of surgery. The operations most commonly associated with this disorder are transurethral resection of the prostate and hysteroscopic uterine submucosal resection. The amount of water absorbed depends upon the hydrostatic pressure of the irrigating fluid, the number and size of the venous sinuses opened, the duration of surgery, and the venous pressure at the irrigant–blood interface. It can also be caused by anaesthetists giving excessive glucose-containing intravenous fluids.

The signs and symptoms are listed below:

- Confusion
- Vomiting
- Restlessness
- Blurred vision
- Transient blindness
- Convulsions
- Bradycardia
- Hypotension
- Hypertension
- Pulmonary oedema
- Asystole.

The tests to confirm the diagnosis include:

- Haemoglobin
- Haematocrit
- Plasma sodium
- Plasma potassium
- Serum osmolality
- Plasma glycine
- Plasma ammonia.

The low haemoglobin, low osmolality, and low plasma sodium confirm the diagnosis. If the sodium is below 120 mmol/l serious signs and symptoms can occur. The glycine and ammonia level results will be delayed but are confirmatory of the diagnosis.

KEYWORDS: WATER INTOXICATION

8. Write a short essay on paracetamol intoxication.

The maximum therapeutic dosage of paracetamol for an average adult is 4 g/24 h. Doses exceeding 8 g are likely to exceed the ability of hepatic glutathione to conjugate the toxic metabolites of paracetamol and cause paracetamol poisoning. Nausea may be the only symptom. The severity of the poisoning is judged on the history and the amount of ingested paracetamol but more importantly on the blood level of paracetamol with the time of the sample and the time of ingestion of paracetamol taken into account. A single measurement of plasma paracetamol concentration related to the time of ingestion is commonly used to enter a paracetamol poisoning nomogram. Plasma concentrations exceeding 250 mg/l at 4 hours or 50 mg/l at 12 hours, for example are associated with severe liver injury and a subsequent mortality rate of 10–20%.

Immediate actions should be taken to minimise injury and these are categorised as follows:

Limit absorption

- Encourage emesis if the patient is seen within 4 hours of ingestion of paracetamol. Ipecacuanha emetic mixture may be used to induce vomiting.
- Consider gastric emptying and lavage if the patient is seen within 2 hours.
- Active adsorbent may be used such as active charcoal.

Remove from blood

In severe cases the following are considered:

- Charcoal haemoperfusion
- Haemodialysis.

Reduce hepatotoxicity

- Acetylcysteine is the specific antidote, and is the mainstay of therapy. It is very effective in protecting the liver provided it is given within the first 12 hours. It is still effective, however, up to and possibly beyond 24 hours.
- Methionine is an alternative therapy. It is used in cases of known allergy to acetylcysteine. It is also used for a prehospital treatment, or when intravenous excess is difficult, as it is given orally.
- The use of steroids is controversial.

KEYWORDS: PARACETAMOL INTOXICATION

Criteria for considering liver transplant includes persistent encephalopathy (grade 3 or 4), blood pH < 7.3, international normalised ratio > 6.5 and creatinine levels > 300 micromol/l.

KEYWORDS: PARACETAMOL INTOXICATION

9. Describe how brain-stem death is confirmed.

It is essential that certain preconditions and exclusions are fulfilled before a diagnosis of brain-stem death can be made.

Preconditions

- Apnoeic coma (unresponsive and on a ventilator, with no spontaneous respiratory efforts).
- Irremediable structural brain damage of known cause.

Exclusions

- Poisons, sedative drugs, and neuromuscular blocking agents.
- Hypothermia (central body temperature should be >35°C).
- Metabolic or endocrine disturbances (no profound abnormality of plasma electrolytes, acid-base balance, or blood glucose levels).

Assessment of brain-stem function

- It is necessary to establish that all brain-stem reflexes are absent: pupillary, corneal, oculocephalic, vestibulo-ocular, gag, and cough.
- There should be no motor response within the cranial nerve territory to painful stimuli applied centrally or peripherally.
- Spontaneous respiration should be absent. This test is crucial to the diagnosis of brain-stem death.

In the UK, it is not necessary to perform tests such as EEG and carotid angiography for confirmation of brain-stem death.

Tests should be performed

- By two doctors once the preconditions have been met. Diagnosis should not normally be considered until at least six hours after the onset of coma or if anoxia or cardiac arrest was the cause of the coma (particularly in children), until 24 hours after the circulation has been restored.
- By two medical practitioners of adequate experience. One should be a consultant, the other another consultant or a doctor registered for more than five years; neither should be a member of the transplant team.
- On two separate occasions, the interval between the two being agreed by all the staff involved.

KEYWORDS: BRAIN-STEM DEATH

10. Compare and contrast the use of systemic opioids and thoracic epidural bupivacaine administration for postoperative analgesia following elective surgery for abdominal aortic aneurysm surgery.

Systemic opioids

These may be given by the oral, intramuscular, intravenous, or subcutaneous routes by intermittent injections, PCA, or continuous infusions.

Advantages

- Less technical skill required; can be administered by nursing staff.
- Safe to run for many days.
- Does not necessarily require HDU/ITU facilities.
- Avoids complications specific to regional analgesia, for example dural headache.
- Cheap.

Disadvantages

- Less effective analgesia.
- Sedation.
- Respiratory depression, cough suppression with basal atelectasis.
- Reduced GIT motility and constipation.
- Nausea and vomiting.
- Tolerance.
- Risk of addiction (long-term).

Thoracic epidurals

Advantages

- Generally produce excellent local analgesia without systemic side effects.
- Allow patient to breathe deeply and cough effectively.

Disadvantages

- Technically difficult with a risk of trauma to the spinal cord.
- All the possible problems associated with siting an epidural catheter such as infection, inadvertent dural puncture, haematoma formation, anterior spinal artery syndrome, and adhesive arachnoiditis.
- Problems associated with the use of local anaesthetics such as hypotension, high blocks, and total spinal block.
- Problems associated with epidural opioids such as respiratory depression, pruritis, nausea and vomiting, and urinary retention.
- Ineffective in a small proportion of patients owing to incomplete block.

KEYWORDS: OPIOIDS; BUPIVACAINE; POSTOPERATIVE ANALGESIA

- May require High Dependency Unit care depending on local policy.
- A doctor is currently often required to make up epidural infusions or give boluses; doctor unavailability may delay provision of analgesia.
- Expensive.

KEYWORDS: OPIOIDS; BUPIVACAINE; POSTOPERATIVE ANALGESIA

11. Outline the intraoperative problems that may occur during elective surgery for an infrarenal abdominal aortic aneurysm.

Patients presenting for aortic aneurysmal surgery constitute a high risk surgical group. The majority are elderly, smokers, and many have co-existing diseases such as ischaemic heart disease, hypertension, carotid and cerebrovascular disease, renal impairment, diabetes mellitus, and chronic pulmonary disease.

Intraoperative problems

- Acute haemodynamic changes, associated with induction, laryngoscopy and intubation, cross-clamping, unclamping, and emergence.
- Hypoperfusion of vital organs, associated with underlying atherosclerosis, cross-clamping.
- Severe increases in left ventricular afterload from cross-clamping.
- Major blood loss, coagulopathies, massive transfusion, and attendant complications.
- Acid-base disturbances.
- Hypothermia, associated with prolonged surgery and evaporative losses.

Effects of cross-clamping the abdominal aorta

- Acute increase in left ventricular afterload can result in hypertension, cardiac ischaemia, acute left ventricular failure.
- Renal ischaemia can occur even with infrarenal clamping; surgery may result in arterial emboli to the kidneys; patients with pre-existing renal disease are at a higher risk of developing perioperative acute renal failure.
- Interruption of spinal cord perfusion can result in paraplegia.
- Intestinal ischaemia can result in intestinal colitis.

Effects of removal of aortic cross-clamp

- Decrease in systemic vascular resistance leads to hypotension.
- Washout of lactate and accumulated metabolites in the ischaemic limbs produces an acute metabolic acidosis.

NB. The effects of cross-clamp removal can be minimised by releasing the clamp slowly and by fluid loading before the clamp comes off.

The intraoperative problems can be minimised by identification and quantification of patients at risk of perioperative cardiac morbidity; institution of appropriate treatment to optimise patients prior to surgery; careful attention to anaesthetic technique; meticulous attention to fluid

KEYWORDS: ABDOMINAL AORTIC ANEURYSM

management aided by invasive pressure monitoring, measurement of urinary volumes, acid-base and electrolyte balance; an experienced vascular surgeon!

KEYWORDS: ABDOMINAL AORTIC ANEURYSM

12. List the nerves blocked during an ankle block and indicate where they may be blocked. What are the complications associated with this block?

The nerves blocked during an ankle block are:

- *Deep peroneal nerve.* This is blocked by injecting around the dorsalis pedis artery, between the tendons of tibialis anterior and extensor hallucis longus muscles.
- *Superficial peroneal nerve.* This is blocked by infiltrating local anaesthetic superficially under the skin in a fan shape, superior to the lateral malleolus and round to the anterior border of the tibia.
- *Sural nerve.* This is blocked at the same time as the superficial peroneal nerve. If this proves ineffective, a further distal infiltration between the lateral malleolus and the calcaneus will usually prove effective.
- *Tibial nerve.* This is blocked by injecting just anterolateral to the posterior tibial artery, posterior to the medial malleolus.
- *Saphenous nerve.* This is blocked by infiltrating in a superficial, subcutaneous fan shape, superior to the medial malleolus.

The problems with this block are:

- It may take 45 minutes before being fully effective.
- It has a significant failure rate.
- There is a risk of intravascular injection.
- It involves four injections, which may be unacceptable to the patient.
- There are local anaesthetic complications and toxicity.

KEYWORDS: ANKLE BLOCK

Index by Keywords

The entry location is paper followed by question number; for example, D11 is paper D, question 11.

abdominal aortic aneurysm I11
abscess, arm C5
acute respiratory distress syndrome C10
AIDS I5
    perioperative management D11
air embolism D5
airway obstruction, upper E12
ambulance transfer F12
analgesia E2, G6, I10
anaphylaxis B8
anatomy
    antecubital fossa C6
    diaphragm C6, 1/G4
    larynx F9, I3
    oesophagus E7
    rib B3
    trachea A9
ankle block I12
ankylosing spondylitis A8
antecubital fossa anatomy C6
antibiotics in ICU H3
anticoagulation H10
anticonvulsants B7
aortic aneurysm I11
ARDS C10
arm abscess C5
arrhythmias, cardiac F5
audit A10

bicarbonate G12
blood flow, cerebral D6
blood transfusion
    complications E9
    filters D7
brachial plexus block H9
brain damage D3
brain-stem death F2, I9
breast carcinoma A6
breathing system filters D7
bronchoscopy C9, F10

bupivacaine I10
burns C1

caesarean section G7
capnography G3
cardiac arrest G8, G12
cardiac arrhythmias F5
cardiac see also heart
catheter, pulmonary artery flotation E5
CEMD A10
central venous pressure B2
cerebral blood flow D6
chest drain G9
children
    eye injury H4
    premedication E8
    squint B12
    stridor E12
chronic pain management A6
coma D3
CVP B2
cystic fibrosis C3

dantrolene I1
day-care surgery E11, F6, I2
    discharge E11
decontamination A5, G9
deep venous thrombosis E1
diaphragm
    anatomy G4
    function D1
discectomy G5
discharge
    from day-surgery unit E11, I2
    from recovery unit A7
disinfection A5
distribution curve, normal D10
drug
    abuse, intravenous I6
    addiction C5
DVT E1

159

eclampsia
  management F1
  warning signs B7
elderly patients F8
embolism
  air D5
  fat H5
  pulmonary C8
emergency anaesthesia I16
epidural infusion filters D7
epistaxis F8
equipment, sterilisation A5
ethical research E3
extravasation D12
eye injury, penetrating H4

fat embolism H5
fibreoptic intubation B10
filters D7
foreign body inhalation F10

Glasgow Coma Scale D3
Gram negative infections D8

haemodialysis F7
haemofiltration F7
head injury D3, E10
heart
  block G8
  valve H10
  see also cardiac
hepatitis B G9
herniorrhaphy, inguinal E11
heroin addiction C5
HIV D11, I5
hyperpyrexia, malignant I1
hypertension, pregnancy-induced A1
hyperthermia, malignant E4
hypotensive anaesthesia H2
hypothermia B11, G2
hypoxaemia B1, H12

infection, Gram negative D8
infusion, target-controlled B4
inguinal herniorrhaphy E11, I2
intensive care unit D8, H3, H8
interpleural block G11
intra-arterial thiopentone C6
intracranial pressure B9
intravenous anaesthesia, total B4
intravenous drug abuse I6
intubation
  failed G7
  fibreoptic B10

teeth and C7

laparoscopy D4
laryngoscopy F9
larynx B10
  anatomy F9, I3
  laser surgery F11
laser surgery F11
letter writing E4
lumbar discectomy G5

magnesium therapy C4
malignant hyperpyrexia I1
malignant hyperthermia E4
maternal deaths A10
monitoring problems F12
MRI scan E6
muscle relaxants H8
muscular dystrophies F4
myotonia F4

nausea and vomiting G1
NCEPOD A10
neonatal premedication E8
nerve supply to larynx I3
neurosurgery unit F12
  referral E10
normal distribution curve D10
nosocomial pneumonia I5

obesity A4, F6
obstetrics B7, F1, G7, H11
oesophagoscopy E7
oesophagus, anatomy E7
opioids I10
organ
  donation F2
  transplant G10
orthopaedics G5

pacemakers B6
pacing, temporary G8
pain management G6
  chronic A6
  postoperative E2, I10
paracetamol intoxication I8
parametric/non-parametric tests A2
PEEP F3
pleural cavity injection G11
pneumonia, nosocomial I5
pneumothorax C2, G9
PONV G1
porphyria A3
position of patient, prone C12, G5

positive end expiratory pressure F3
postoperative analgesia E2, I10
postoperative hypoxaemia B1
postoperative nausea and vomiting G1
postpartum haemorrhage H11
pregnancy-induced hypertension A1
premedication for children E8
probability A2
prone position C12, G5
prostate, transurethral resection A12
prosthetic heart valve H10
pulmonary artery flotation catheter E5
pulmonary embolism C8
pulse oximetry C11

recovery unit care A7
red cell storage E9
referral of patient to neurosurgical unit
  E10
research, ethical E3
respiratory distress syndrome, acute
C10
respiratory failure I5
rheumatoid arthritis D2
rib
  anatomy, first B3
  fracture G6
  metastasis A6

sedation H8
septic shock D8
smoking H7
sodium bicarbonate G12
squint B12

statistics A2, D10
stellate ganglion block A11, H1
sterilisation of equipment A5
stress ulcers B5
stridor in children E12
subclavian venepuncture E5
suxamethonium H6

tachycardia I4
target-controlled infusion B4
teeth C7
thiopentone
  extravasation D12
  intra-arterial C6
thoracotomy E2
thyroidectomy D9
TIVA B4
total intravenous anaesthesia B4
trachea, anatomy A9
tracheostomy A9
transfer to neurosurgery F12
transurethral resection of prostate A12
TURP A12

ulcers, stress B5
upper airway obstruction E12

vancomycin H3
venepuncture, subclavian E5
ventricular tachycardia I4
vocal cords F9
vomiting G1

water intoxication I7